Digestive
Diseases and
Disorders
SOURCEBOOK

Digestive
Diseases and
Disorders
SOURCEBOOK

*Basic Consumer Health Information about Diseases
and Disorders that Impact the Upper and Lower
Digestive System, Including Celiac Disease,
Constipation, Crohn's Disease, Cyclic Vomiting
Syndrome, Diarrhea, Diverticulosis and
Diverticulitis, Gallstones, Heartburn, Hemorrhoids,
Hernias, Indigestion (Dyspepsia), Irritable Bowel
Syndrome, Lactose Intolerance, Ulcers, and More;
Along with Information about Medications and
Other Treatments, Tips for Maintaining a Healthy
Digestive Tract, a Glossary, and Directory of
Digestive Diseases Organizations*

Edited by
Karen Bellenir

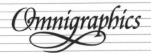

Omnigraphics

615 Griswold • Detroit, MI 48226

BS

Bibliographic Note

Because this page cannot legibly accommodate all the copyright notices, the Bibliographic Note portion of the Preface constitutes an extension of the copyright notice.

Beginning with books published in 1999, each new volume of the *Health Reference Series* will be individually titled and called a "First Edition." Subsequent updates will carry sequential edition numbers. To help avoid confusion and to provide maximum flexibility in our ability to respond to informational needs, the practice of consecutively numbering each volume will be discontinued.

Edited by Karen Bellenir

Health Reference Series

Karen Bellenir, *Series Editor*
Peter D. Dresser, *Managing Editor*
Joan Margeson, *Research Associate*
Dawn Matthews, *Verification Assistant*
Margaret Mary Missar, *Research Coordinator*
Jenifer Swanson, *Research Associate*

Omnigraphics, Inc.

Matthew P. Barbour, *Vice President, Operations*
Laurie Lanzen Harris, *Vice President, Editorial Director*
Kevin Hayes, *Production Coordinator*
Thomas J. Murphy, *Vice President, Finance and Comptroller*
Peter E. Ruffner, *Senior Vice President*
Jane J. Steele, *Marketing Consultant*

Frederick G. Ruffner, Jr., Publisher

© 2000, Omnigraphics, Inc.

Library of Congress Cataloging-in-Publication Data

Digestive diseases and disorders sourcebook : basic consumer health information about diseases and disorders that impact the upper and lower digestive system . . . / edited by Karen Bellenir. — 1st ed.
    p. ; cm. — (Health reference series)
Includes bibliographical references and index.
ISBN 0-7808-0327-2 (library binding : alk. paper)
    1. Gastrointestinal system—Diseases—Popular Works. I. Bellenir, Karen. II. Health reference series (Unnumbered)
[DNLM: 1. Digestive System Diseases—Popular Works. 2. Digestive System Diseases—Resources Guides. 3. Health Education—Popular Works. 4. Health Education—Resource Guides. WI 39 D572 2000]
RC816.D544 2000
816.3—dc21   99-045761

∞

This book is printed on acid-free paper meeting the ANSI Z39.48 Standard. The infinity symbol that appears above indicates that the paper in this book meets that standard.

Printed in the United States

9/5/0~

Table of Contents

Part III: Additional Help and Information

Preface

About this Book

An estimated 62 million Americans are diagnosed with digestive disorders every year. Some digestive diseases are sudden and self-limiting; others can be chronic, debilitating, and even life-threatening. The prevalence of most digestive diseases increases with age, and women are more likely to report a digestive condition than are men. Combined, digestive diseases have an enormous impact. For example, every year digestive diseases:

- result in nearly 200 million sick days and 16.9 million days lost from school
- account for 50 million visits to physicians
- are responsible for 10 million hospitalizations
- cause 200,000 deaths

This *Sourcebook* offers basic information for the layperson about common disorders of the upper and lower digestive tract, including celiac disease, constipation, Crohn's disease, cyclic vomiting syndrome, diarrhea, diverticulosis and diverticulitis, gallstones, heartburn, hemorrhoids, hernias, indigestion (dyspepsia), irritable bowel syndrome, lactose intolerance, ulcers, and more. Tips for maintaining a healthy digestive tract, a glossary of important terms, and a directory of digestive diseases organizations are also provided.

How to Use This Book

This book is divided into parts and chapters. Parts focus on broad areas of interest. Chapters are devoted to single topics within a part.

Part I: Maintaining a Healthy Digestive Tract offers a description of the digestive tract, a summary of facts and statistics about digestive diseases, an explanation of common diagnostic tests, and tips for disease prevention.

Part II: Digestive Diseases and Functional Disorders presents information on about 26 different diseases of the digestive system and other disorders of digestive functioning. The chapters are ordered alphabetically to ensure ease of access.

Part III: Additional Help and Information provides a glossary of terms related to digestive diseases and a directory of organizations able to provide further assistance.

Bibliographic Note

This volume contains documents and excerpts from publications issued by the following government agencies: National Digestive Diseases Information Clearinghouse (NDIC), National Institute of Diabetes and Digestive and Kidney Diseases (NIDDK), and the U.S. Food and Drug Administration (FDA).

In addition, this volume contains copyrighted articles from the American College of Surgeons, Cyclic Vomiting Syndrome Association, Intestinal Disease Foundation, Inc., Tap Pharmaceuticals, Inc., and the United Ostomy Association.

Full citation information is provided on the first page of each chapter. Every effort has been made to secure all necessary rights to reprint the copyrighted material. If any omissions have been made, please contact Omnigraphics to make corrections for future editions.

Acknowledgements

In addition to the organizations listed above, special thanks are due to document engineer Bruce Bellenir, researchers Jenifer Swanson and Joan Margeson, verification assistant Dawn Matthews, and permissions specialist Maria Franklin.

Note from the Editor

This book is part of Omnigraphics' *Health Reference Series*. The series provides basic information about a broad range of medical concerns. It is not intended to serve as a tool for diagnosing illness, in prescribing treatments, or as a substitute for the physician/patient relationship. All persons concerned about medical symptoms or the possibility of disease are encouraged to seek professional care from an appropriate health care provider.

Our Advisory Board

The *Health Reference Series* is reviewed by an Advisory Board comprised of librarians from public, academic, and medical libraries. We would like to thank the following board members for providing guidance to the development of this series:

Nancy Bulgarelli, William Beaumont Hospital Library, Royal Oak, MI

Karen Imarasio, Bloomfield Township Public Library, Bloomfield Township, MI

Karen Morgan, Mardigian Library, University of Michigan-Dearborn, Dearborn, MI

Rosemary Orlando, St. Clair Shores Public Library, St. Clair Shores, MI

Health Reference Series *Update Policy*

The inaugural book in the *Health Reference Series* was the first edition of *Cancer Sourcebook* published in 1992. Since then, the *Series* has been enthusiastically received by librarians and in the medical community. In order to maintain the standard of providing high-quality health information for the lay person, the editorial staff at Omnigraphics felt it was necessary to implement a policy of updating volumes when warranted.

Medical researchers have been making tremendous strides, and the challenge to stay current with the most recent advances is one our editors take seriously. Each decision to update a volume will be made on an individual basis. Some of the considerations will include how much new information is available and the feedback we receive from people who use the books. If there's a topic you would like to see added to the update list, or an area of medical concern you feel has not been adequately addressed, please write to:

Editor
Health Reference Series
Omnigraphics, Inc.
615 Griswold
Detroit, MI 48226

The commitment to providing on-going coverage of important medical developments has also led to some technical changes in the *Health Reference Series*. Beginning with books published in 1999, each new volume will be individually titled and called a "First Edition." Subsequent updates will carry sequential edition numbers. To help avoid confusion and to provide maximum flexibility in our ability to respond to informational needs, the practice of consecutively numbering each volume will be discontinued.

Part One

Maintaining a Healthy Digestive Tract

Chapter 1

Your Digestive System and How It Works

The digestive system is a series of hollow organs joined in a long, twisting tube from the mouth to the anus (see Figure 1.1). Inside this tube is a lining called the mucosa. In the mouth, stomach, and small intestine, the mucosa contains tiny glands that produce juices to help digest food.

There are also two solid digestive organs, the liver and the pancreas, which produce juices that reach the intestine through small tubes. In addition, parts of other organ systems (for instance, nerves and blood) play a major role in the digestive system.

Why Is Digestion Important?

When we eat such things as bread, meat, and vegetables, they are not in a form that the body can use as nourishment. Our food and drink must be changed into smaller molecules of nutrients before they can be absorbed into the blood and carried to cells throughout the body. Digestion is the process by which food and drink are broken down into their smallest parts so that the body can use them to build and nourish cells and to provide energy.

How Is Food Digested?

Digestion involves the mixing of food, its movement through the digestive tract, and chemical breakdown of the large molecules of food

National Institute of Diabetes and Digestive and Kidney Diseases (NIDDK), National Institutes of Health, NIH Pub. No. 97-2681, updated January 1999.

3

into smaller molecules. Digestion begins in the mouth, when we chew and swallow, and is completed in the small intestine. The chemical process varies somewhat for different kinds of food.

Movement of Food through the System

The large, hollow organs of the digestive system contain muscle that enables their walls to move. The movement of organ walls can propel food and liquid and also can mix the contents within each organ. Typical movement of the esophagus, stomach, and intestine is called peristalsis. The action of peristalsis looks like an ocean wave

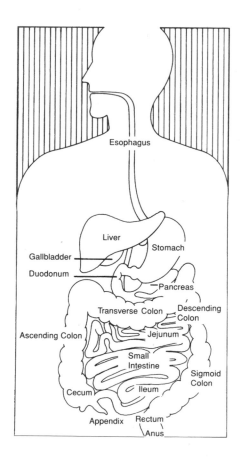

Figure 1.1. *The Digestive System*

moving through the muscle. The muscle of the organ produces a narrowing and then propels the narrowed portion slowly down the length of the organ. These waves of narrowing push the food and fluid in front of them through each hollow organ.

The first major muscle movement occurs when food or liquid is swallowed. Although we are able to start swallowing by choice, once the swallow begins, it becomes involuntary and proceeds under the control of the nerves.

The esophagus is the organ into which the swallowed food is pushed. It connects the throat above with the stomach below. At the junction of the esophagus and stomach, there is a ringlike valve closing the passage between the two organs. However, as the food approaches the closed ring, the surrounding muscles relax and allow the food to pass.

The food then enters the stomach, which has three mechanical tasks to do. First, the stomach must store the swallowed food and liquid. This requires the muscle of the upper part of the stomach to relax and accept large volumes of swallowed material. The second job is to mix up the food, liquid, and digestive juice produced by the stomach. The lower part of the stomach mixes these materials by its muscle action. The third task of the stomach is to empty its contents slowly into the small intestine.

Several factors affect emptying of the stomach, including the nature of the food (mainly its fat and protein content) and the degree of muscle action of the emptying stomach and the next organ to receive the stomach contents (the small intestine). As the food is digested in the small intestine and dissolved into the juices from the pancreas, liver, and intestine, the contents of the intestine are mixed and pushed forward to allow further digestion.

Finally, all of the digested nutrients are absorbed through the intestinal walls. The waste products of this process include undigested parts of the food, known as fiber, and older cells that have been shed from the mucosa. These materials are propelled into the colon, where they remain, usually for a day or two, until the feces are expelled by a bowel movement.

Production of Digestive Juices

Glands of the digestive system are crucial to the process of digestion. They produce both the juices that break down the food and the hormones that help to control the process.

The glands that act first are in the mouth—the salivary glands. Saliva produced by these glands contains an enzyme that begins to digest the starch from food into smaller molecules.

The next set of digestive glands is in the stomach lining. They produce stomach acid and an enzyme that digests protein. One of the unsolved puzzles of the digestive system is why the acid juice of the stomach does not dissolve the tissue of the stomach itself. In most people, the stomach mucosa is able to resist the juice, although food and other tissues of the body cannot.

After the stomach empties the food and its juice into the small intestine, the juices of two other digestive organs mix with the food to continue the process of digestion. One of these organs is the pancreas. It produces a juice that contains a wide array of enzymes to break down the carbohydrates, fat, and protein in our food. Other enzymes that are active in the process come from glands in the wall of the intestine or even a part of that wall.

The liver produces yet another digestive juice—bile. The bile is stored between meals in the gallbladder. At mealtime, it is squeezed out of the gallbladder into the bile ducts to reach the intestine and mix with the fat in our food. The bile acids dissolve the fat into the watery contents of the intestine, much like detergents that dissolve grease from a frying pan. After the fat is dissolved, it is digested by enzymes from the pancreas and the lining of the intestine.

Absorption and Transport of Nutrients

Digested molecules of food, as well as water and minerals from the diet, are absorbed from the cavity of the upper small intestine. The absorbed materials cross the mucosa into the blood, mainly, and are carried off in the bloodstream to other parts of the body for storage or further chemical change. As noted above, this part of the process varies with different types of nutrients.

Carbohydrates. An average American adult eats about half a pound of carbohydrate each day. Some of our most common foods contain mostly carbohydrates. Examples are bread, potatoes, pastries, candy, rice, spaghetti, fruits, and vegetables. Many of these foods contain both starch, which can be digested, and fiber, which the body cannot digest.

The digestible carbohydrates are broken into simpler molecules by enzymes in the saliva, in juice produced by the pancreas, and in the lining of the small intestine. Starch is digested in two steps: First, an enzyme in the saliva and pancreatic juice breaks the starch into molecules called maltose; then an enzyme in the lining of the small intestine (maltase) splits the maltose into glucose molecules that can be absorbed into the blood. Glucose is carried through the bloodstream to the liver, where it is stored or used to provide energy for the work of the body.

Table sugar is another carbohydrate that must be digested to be useful. An enzyme in the lining of the small intestine digests table sugar into glucose and fructose, each of which can be absorbed from the intestinal cavity into the blood. Milk contains yet another type of sugar, lactose, which is changed into absorbable molecules by an enzyme called lactase, also found in the intestinal lining.

Protein. Foods such as meat, eggs, and beans consist of giant molecules of protein that must be digested by enzymes before they can be used to build and repair body tissues. An enzyme in the juice of the stomach starts the digestion of swallowed protein. Further digestion of the protein is completed in the small intestine. Here, several enzymes from the pancreatic juice and the lining of the intestine carry out the breakdown of huge protein molecules into small molecules called amino acids. These small molecules can be absorbed from the hollow of the small intestine into the blood and then be carried to all parts of the body to build the walls and other parts of cells.

Fats. Fat molecules are a rich source of energy for the body. The first step in digestion of a fat such as butter is to dissolve it into the watery content of the intestinal cavity. The bile acids produced by the liver act as natural detergents to dissolve fat in water and allow the enzymes to break the large fat molecules into smaller molecules, some of which are fatty acids and cholesterol. The bile acids combine with the fatty acids and cholesterol and help these molecules to move into the cells of the mucosa. In these cells the small molecules are formed back into large molecules, most of which pass into vessels (called lymphatics) near the intestine. These small vessels carry the reformed fat to the veins of the chest, and the blood carries the fat to storage depots in different parts of the body.

Vitamins. Another vital part of our food that is absorbed from the small intestine is the class of chemicals we call vitamins. There are two different types of vitamins, classified by the fluid in which they can be dissolved: water-soluble vitamins (all the B vitamins and vitamin C) and fat-soluble vitamins (vitamins A, D, and K).

7

Water and Salt. Most of the material absorbed from the cavity of the small intestine is water in which salt is dissolved. The salt and water come from the food and liquid we swallow and the juices secreted by the many digestive glands. In a healthy adult, more than a gallon of water containing over an ounce of salt is absorbed from the intestine every 24 hours.

How Is the Digestive Process Controlled?

Hormone Regulators

A fascinating feature of the digestive system is that it contains its own regulators. The major hormones that control the functions of the digestive system are produced and released by cells in the mucosa of the stomach and small intestine. These hormones are released into the blood of the digestive tract, travel back to the heart and through the arteries, and return to the digestive system, where they stimulate digestive juices and cause organ movement. The hormones that control digestion are gastrin, secretin, and cholecystokinin (CCK):

- Gastrin causes the stomach to produce an acid for dissolving and digesting some foods. It is also necessary for the normal growth of the lining of the stomach, small intestine, and colon.

- Secretin causes the pancreas to send out a digestive juice that is rich in bicarbonate. It stimulates the stomach to produce pepsin, an enzyme that digests protein, and it also stimulates the liver to produce bile.

- CCK causes the pancreas to grow and to produce the enzymes of pancreatic juice, and it causes the gallbladder to empty.

Nerve Regulators

Two types of nerves help to control the action of the digestive system. Extrinsic (outside) nerves come to the digestive organs from the unconscious part of the brain or from the spinal cord. They release a chemical called acetylcholine and another called adrenaline. Acetylcholine causes the muscle of the digestive organs to squeeze with more force and increase the "push" of food and juice through the digestive tract. Acetylcholine also causes the stomach and pancreas to produce more digestive juice. Adrenaline relaxes the muscle of the stomach and intestine and decreases the flow of blood to these organs.

Even more important, though, are the intrinsic (inside) nerves, which make up a very dense network embedded in the walls of the esophagus, stomach, small intestine, and colon. The intrinsic nerves are triggered to act when the walls of the hollow organs are stretched by food. They release many different substances that speed up or delay the movement of food and the production of juices by the digestive organs.

Chapter 2

Facts and Fallacies about Digestive Diseases

Introduction

Researchers have only recently begun to understand the many, often complex, diseases that affect the digestive system. Accordingly, people are gradually replacing folklore, old wives' tales, and rumors about the causes and treatments of digestive diseases with accurate, up-to-date information. But misunderstandings still exist, and, while some folklore is harmless, some can be dangerous if it keeps a person from correctly preventing or treating an illness. Listed below are some common misconceptions (fallacies), about digestive diseases, followed by the facts as professionals understand them today.

True or False?

Ulcers: *Spicy food and stress cause stomach ulcers.*

False. The truth is, almost all stomach ulcers are caused either by infection with a bacterium called *Helicobacter pylori (H. pylori)* or by use of pain medications such as aspirin, ibuprofen, or naproxen, the so-called nonsteroidal anti-inflammatory drugs (NSAIDs). Most *H. pylori*-related ulcers can be cured with antibiotics. NSAID-induced ulcers can be cured with time, stomach-protective medications, antacids, and avoidance of NSAIDs. Spicy food and stress may aggravate ulcer symptoms in some people, but they do not cause ulcers.

National Institute of Diabetes and Digestive and Kidney Diseases (NIDDK), NIH Pub. No. 99-2673, January 1999.

11

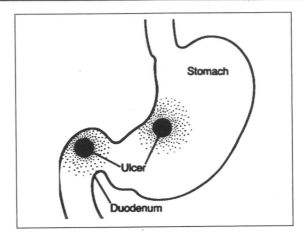

Figure 2.1. Peptic ulcers are sores in the lining of the stomach or duodenum.

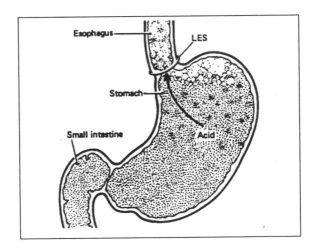

Figure 2.2. Heartburn occurs when the lower esophageal sphincter (called the LES), located at the junction of the esophagus and the stomach, either relaxes inappropriately or is very weak. This allows the highly acidic contents of the stomach to back up into the esophagus.

Heartburn: Smoking a cigarette helps relieve heartburn.

False. Actually, cigarette smoking contributes to heartburn. Heartburn occurs when the lower esophageal sphincter (LES)—a muscle between the esophagus and stomach—relaxes, allowing the acidic contents of the stomach to splash back into the esophagus. Cigarette smoking causes the LES to relax.

Celiac Disease: Celiac disease is a rare childhood disease.

False. Celiac disease affects children and adults. At least 1 in 1,000 people and, in some populations, 1 in 200 people have celiac disease. Most often, celiac disease first causes symptoms during childhood, usually diarrhea, growth failure, and failure to thrive. But the disease can also first cause symptoms in adults. These symptoms may be vague and therefore attributed to other conditions. Symptoms can include bloating, diarrhea, abdominal pain, skin rash, anemia, and thinning of the bones (osteoporosis). Celiac disease may cause such nonspecific symptoms for several years before being correctly diagnosed and treated.

People with celiac disease should not eat any foods containing gluten, a protein in wheat, rye, barley, and possibly oats, regardless of whether or not they have symptoms. In these people, gluten destroys part of the lining of the small intestine, which interferes with the absorption of nutrients. The damage can occur from even a small amount of gluten, and not everyone has symptoms of damage.

Bowel Regularity: Bowel regularity means a bowel movement every day.

False. The frequency of bowel movements among normal, healthy people varies from three a day to three a week, and perfectly healthy people may fall outside both ends of this range.

Constipation: Habitual use of enemas to treat constipation is harmless.

False. The truth is, habitual use of enemas is not harmless. Over time, enemas can impair the natural muscle action of the intestines, leaving them unable to function normally. An ongoing need for enemas is not normal; you should see a doctor if you find yourself relying on them or any other medication to have a bowel movement.

Irritable Bowel Syndrome: Irritable bowel syndrome is a disease.

False. Irritable bowel syndrome is not a disease. It is a functional disorder, which means that there is a problem in how the muscles in the intestines work. Irritable bowel syndrome is characterized by gas, abdominal pain, and diarrhea or constipation, or both. Although the syndrome can cause considerable pain and discomfort, it does not damage the digestive tract as diseases do. Also, irritable bowel syndrome does not lead to more serious digestive diseases later.

Diverticulosis: Diverticulosis is an uncommon and serious problem.

False. Actually, the majority of Americans over age 60 have diverticulosis, but only a small percentage have symptoms or complications. Diverticulosis is a condition in which little sacs—or out-pouchings—called diverticula, develop in the wall of the colon. These tend to appear and increase in number with age. Most people do not have symptoms and would not know that they had diverticula unless x-ray or intestinal examination were done. Less than 10 percent of people with diverticulosis ever develop complications such as infection (diverticulitis), bleeding, or perforation of the colon.

Inflammatory Bowel Disease: Inflammatory bowel disease is caused by psychological problems.

False. Inflammatory bowel disease is the general name for two diseases that cause inflammation in the intestines, Crohn's disease and ulcerative colitis. The cause of the disease is unknown, but researchers speculate that it may be a virus or bacteria interacting with the body's immune system. There is no evidence to support the theory that inflammatory bowel disease is caused by tension, anxiety, or other psychological factors or disorders.

Cirrhosis: Cirrhosis is only caused by alcoholism.

False. Alcoholism is just one of many causes of cirrhosis. Cirrhosis is scarring and decreased function of the liver. In the United States, alcohol causes less than one-half of cirrhosis cases. The remaining cases are from other diseases that cause liver damage. For example, in children, cirrhosis may result from cystic fibrosis, alpha-1 antitrypsin deficiency, biliary atresia, glycogen storage disease, and other rare diseases. In adults, cirrhosis may be caused by hepatitis B or C, primary biliary cirrhosis, diseases of abnormal storage of metals like iron or copper in the body, severe reactions to prescription drugs, or injury to the ducts that drain bile from the liver.

Ostomy Surgery: After ostomy surgery, men become impotent and women have impaired sexual function and are unable to become pregnant.

False. Ostomy surgery does not, in general, interfere with a person's sexual or reproductive capabilities. Ostomy surgery is a procedure in which the diseased part of the small or large intestine is removed and the remaining intestine is attached to an opening in the abdomen. Although some men who have had radical ostomy surgery for cancer lose the ability to achieve and sustain an erection, most men do not experience impotence, or, if they do, it is temporary. If impotence does occur, a variety of solutions are available. A urologist, a doctor who specializes in such problems, can help find the best solution. In women, ostomy surgery does not damage sexual or reproductive organs, so it does not directly cause sexual problems or sterility. Factors such as pain and the adjustment to a new body image may create some temporary sexual problems, but they can usually be resolved with time and, in some cases, counseling. Unless a woman has had a hysterectomy to remove her uterus, she can still bear children.

Additional Resources

American Liver Foundation
1425 Pompton Avenue
Cedar Grove, NJ 07009
Tel: (800) 465-4837 or (973) 256-2550

Celiac Disease Foundation
13251 Ventura Boulevard, Suite 1
Studio City, CA 91604-1838
Tel: (818) 990-2354

Crohn's & Colitis Foundation of America, Inc.
386 Park Avenue South, 17th Floor
New York, NY 10016-8804
Tel: (800) 932-2423 or (212) 685-3440

Hepatitis Foundation International
30 Sunrise Terrace
Cedar Grove, NJ 07009-1423
Tel: (800) 891-0707 or (973) 239-1035

International Foundation for Functional Gastrointestinal Disorders
P.O. Box 17864
Milwaukee, WI 53217
Tel: (414) 964-1799

National Digestive Diseases Information Clearinghouse
2 Information Way
Bethesda, MD 20892-3570
E-mail: nddic@info.niddk.nih.gov

United Ostomy Association
19772 MacArthur Boulevard, Suite 200
Irvine, CA 92612-2405
Tel: (800) 826-0826 or (949) 660-8624

Chapter 3

Digestive Diseases Statistics

All Digestive Diseases[1]

- Prevalence: 60 to 70 million people affected by all digestive diseases (1985)
- Mortality: 191,000, including deaths from cancer (1985)
- Hospitalizations: 10 million (13 percent of all hospitalization) (1985)
- Diagnostic and therapeutic procedures: 6 million (14 percent of all procedures) (1987)
- Physician office visits: 50 million (1985)
- Disability: 1.4 million people (1987)
- Costs:
  $107 billion (1992)
  $87 billion direct medical costs
  $20 billion indirect costs (e.g., disability and mortality)

Specific Diseases

Abdominal Wall Hernia

- Incidence: 800,000 new cases, including 500,000 inguinal hernias (1985)

National Institute of Diabetes and Digestive and Kidney Diseases (NIDDK), NIH Pub. No. 99-3873, February 1995, updated November 1998.

- Prevalence: 4.5 million people (1988-90)
- Hospitalizations: 640,000 (1980)
- Physician office visits: 2 to 3million (1989-90)
- Prescriptions: 184,000 (1989-90)
- Disability: 550,000people (1983-87)

Chronic Liver Disease and Cirrhosis

- Prevalence: 400,000 people (1976-80)
- Mortality: 26,050 deaths (1987)
- Hospitalizations: 300,000 (1987)
- Physician office visits: 1 million (1985)
- Disability: 112,000 people (1983-87)

Constipation

- Prevalence: 4.4 million people (1983-87)
- Mortality: 29 deaths (1982-85)
- Hospitalizations: 100,000 (1983-87)
- Physician office visits: 2million (1985)
- Prescriptions: 1 million (1985)
- Disability: 13,000 people (1983-87)

Diverticular Disease

- Incidence: 300,000 new cases (1987)
- Prevalence: 2 million people (1983-87)
- Mortality: 3,000 deaths (1985)
- Hospitalizations: 440,000 (1987)
- Physician office visits: 2 million (1987)
- Disability: 112,000 people (1983-87)

Gallstones

- Prevalence: 16 to 22 million people (1976-87)
- Mortality: 2,975 (1985)
- Hospitalizations: 800,000 (1987)
- Physician office visits: 600,000 to 700,000 (1985)
- Prescriptions: 195,000 (1985)
- Surgical procedures: 500,000 cholecystectomies (1987)
- Disability: 48,000 people (1983-87)

Gastritis and Nonulcer Dyspepsia (NUD)

- Incidence:
    Gastritis: 313,000 new cases (1975)
    Chronic NUD: 444,000 new cases (1975)
    Acute NUD: 8.2 million new cases (1988)
- Prevalence:
    Gastritis: 2.7 million people (1988)
    NUD: 5.8 million people (1988)
- Mortality:
    Gastritis: 703 (1980s)
    NUD: 49 (1980s)
- Hospitalizations:
    Gastritis: 600 (1980s)
    NUD: 65,000 (1980s)
- Physician office visits:
    Gastritis: 3 million (1980s)
    NUD: 800,000 (1980s)
- Prescriptions:
    Gastritis: 2 million (1985)
    NUD: 649,000 (1985)
- Disability:
    Gastritis: 34,000 people (1983-87)
    Chronic NUD: 42,000 people (1983-87)

Gastroesophageal Reflux Disease and Related Esophageal Disorders

- Prevalence: 3 to 7 percent of U.S. population (1985)
- Mortality: 1,000 deaths (1984-88)
- Hospitalizations: 1 million (1985)
- Physician office visits: 4 to 5 million (1985)

Hemorrhoids (1983-87)

- Incidence: 1 million new cases
- Prevalence: 10.4 million people
- Mortality: 17 deaths
- Hospitalizations: 316,000
- Physician office visits: 3.5 million

- Prescriptions: 1.5 million
- Disability: 52,000 people

Infectious Diarrhea

- Incidence: 99 million new cases (1980)
- Mortality: 3,100 deaths (1985)
- Hospitalizations: 462,000 to728,000 (1987)
- Physician office visits: 8 to 12 million (1985)
- Prescriptions: 5 to 8 million (1985)

Inflammatory Bowel Disease (1987)

- Incidence: 2 to 6 new cases per 100,000 people
- Prevalence: 300,000 to 500,000 people
- Mortality: Fewer than 1,000 deaths
- Hospitalizations: 100,000 (64 percent for Crohn's disease)
- Physician office visits: 700,000
- Disability: 119,000 people (1983-87)

Irritable Bowel Syndrome

- Prevalence: 5 million people (1987)
- Hospitalizations: 34,000 (1987)
- Physician office visits: 3.5 million (1987)
- Prescriptions: 2.2 million (1985)
- Disability: 400,000 people (1983-87)

Lactose Intolerance[2]

- Prevalence: 30 to 50 million people (1994)

Pancreatitis

- Incidence: Acute: 17 new cases per 100,000 people (1976-88)
- Mortality: 2,700 deaths (1985)
- Hospitalizations:
    Acute: 125,000 (1987)
    Chronic: 20,000 (1987)
- Physician office visits:
    Acute: 911,000 (1987)
    Chronic: 122,000 (1987)

Peptic Ulcer

- Prevalence: 5 million people (1987)
- Mortality: 6,500 deaths (1987)
- Hospitalizations: 630,000 (1987)
- Physician office visits: 3 to 5 million (1985)
- Prescriptions: 2 million (1985)
- Disability: 401,000 people (1983-87)

Viral Hepatitis

- Incidence:
  Hepatitis A: 32,000 new cases (1992)
  Hepatitis B: 200,000 to 300,000 new cases (1990)
  Hepatitis C: 150,000 new cases (1991)
  Hepatitis D: 70,000 new cases (1990)
- Prevalence:
  Hepatitis A: 32 to 38 percent of U.S. population that have any history of disease (1991)

  Hepatitis B: 4 percent of U.S. population that have any history of disease (1990)

  Hepatitis C and D: Not determined
- Mortality: Fewer than 1,000 deaths (1985)
- Hospitalizations: 33,000 (1987)
- Physician office visits: 500,000 (1985)

Additional Data

- Liver Transplants[3]: 3,300 transplants performed (1993)
- Number of gastroenterologists in the United States[4]: 7,493 (1990)

Sources

1. Unless noted, the data in this fact sheet are from:

    Everhart, J.E. (Ed.) *Digestive Diseases in the United States: Epidemiology and Impact.* U.S. Department of Health and Human Services, National Institutes of Health, National Institute of Diabetes and Digestive and Kidney Diseases. Washington, DC: U.S. Government Printing Office, 1994; NIH publication no. 94-1447.

21

The book answers hundreds of questions about the scope and impact of the major infectious, chronic, and malignant digestive diseases. National and special population based data provide information about the prevalence, incidence, medical care, disability, mortality, and research needs regarding specific digestive diseases. The data were compiled primarily from the surveys of the National Center for Health Statistics, supplemented by other federal agencies and private sources.

The book is available for $15 from the National Digestive Diseases Information Clearinghouse at the address and phone number listed below. Please make checks payable to "NDDIC."

2. National Institute of Diabetes and Digestive and Kidney Diseases, National Institutes of Health.

3. United Network for Organ Sharing Scientific Registry.

4. American Medical Association Physician Characteristics and Distribution in the United States, 1992 Ed., Chicago, Illinois: American Medical Association, 1992, p. 20.

Glossary

Data for digestive diseases as a group and for specific diseases are provided in various categories. Data do not exist in all categories for some diseases. Following are definitions of the categories as used in this fact sheet:

Disability: The number of people in a year whose ability to perform major daily activities such as working, housekeeping, and going to school, is limited and reduced over long periods because of a disease.

Hospitalizations: The number of hospitalizations for a disease in a year.

Incidence: The number of new cases of a disease in the U.S. population in a year.

Mortality: The number of deaths resulting from the disease listed as the underlying or primary cause in a year.

Physician office visits: The number of outpatient visits to office-based physicians for a disease in a year.

Prescriptions: The number of prescriptions written annually for medications to treat a specific disease.

Prevalence: The number of people in the United States affected by a disease or diseases in a year.

Procedures: The number of diagnostic and therapeutic procedures performed annually in a hospital setting.

Chapter 4

Diagnostic Tests for Digestive Disorders

This chapter contains patient education information on six diagnostic tests for gastrointestinal disorders:

- Colonoscopy
- Sigmoidoscopy
- Upper Endoscopy
- ERCP (Endoscopic Retrograde Cholangiopancreatography)
- Lower GI (gastrointestinal) series
- Upper GI (gastrointestinal) series

Colonoscopy

Colonoscopy lets the physician look inside your entire large intestine, from the lowest part, the rectum, all the way up through the colon to the lower end of the small intestine. The procedure is used to diagnose the causes of unexplained changes in bowel habits. It is also used to look for early signs of cancer in the colon and rectum. Colonoscopy enables the physician to see inflamed tissue, abnormal growths, ulcers, bleeding, and muscle spasms.

For the procedure, you will lie on your left side on the examining table. You will probably be given pain medication and a mild sedative to keep you comfortable and to help you relax during the exam.

This chapter contains text from the following publications of the National Institute of Diabetes and Digestive and Kidney Diseases (NIDDK): NIH Pub. Nos. 98-4331, 98-4332, 98-4333, 98-4334, 98-4335, 98-4336, June 1998.

The physician will insert a long, flexible, lighted tube into your rectum and slowly guide it into your colon. The tube is called a colonoscope. The scope transmits an image of the inside of the colon, so the physician can carefully examine the lining of the colon. The scope bends, so the physician can move it around the curves of your colon. You may be asked to change position occasionally to help the physician move the scope. The scope also blows air into your colon, which inflates the colon and helps the physician see better.

If anything unusual is in your colon, like a polyp or inflamed tissue, the physician can remove a piece of it using tiny instruments passed through the scope. That tissue (biopsy) is then sent to a lab

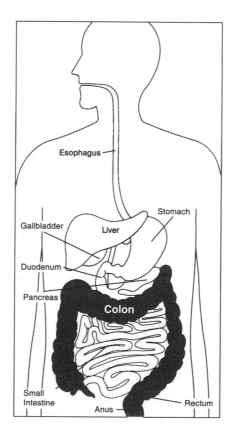

Figure 4.1. *Colonoscopy enables your physician to see inside your entire large intestine.*

for testing. If there is bleeding in the colon, the physician can pass a laser, heater probe, or electrical probe, or inject special medicines, through the scope and use it to stop the bleeding.

Bleeding and puncture of the colon are possible complications of colonoscopy. However, such complications are uncommon.

Colonoscopy takes 30 to 60 minutes. The sedative and pain medicine should keep you from feeling much discomfort during the exam. You will need to remain at the physician's office for 1 to 2 hours until the sedative wears off.

Preparation

Your colon must be completely empty for the colonoscopy to be thorough and safe. To prepare for the procedure you may have to follow a liquid diet for 1 to 3 days beforehand. A liquid diet means fat-free bouillon or broth, Jell-O®, strained fruit juice, water, plain coffee, plain tea, or diet soda. You may need to take laxatives or an enema before the procedure. Also, you must arrange for someone to take you home afterward—you will not be allowed to drive because of the sedatives. Your physician may give you other special instructions.

Sigmoidoscopy

Sigmoidoscopy enables the physician to look at the inside of the large intestine from the rectum through the last part of the colon, called the sigmoid colon. Physicians may use this procedure to find the cause of diarrhea, abdominal pain, or constipation. They also use sigmoidoscopy to look for early signs of cancer in the colon and rectum. With sigmoidoscopy, the physician can see bleeding, inflammation, abnormal growths, and ulcers.

For the procedure, you will lie on your left side on the examining table. The physician will insert a short, flexible, lighted tube into your rectum and slowly guide it into your colon. The tube is called a sigmoidoscope. The scope transmits an image of the inside of the rectum and colon, so the physician can carefully examine the lining of these organs. The scope also blows air into these organs, which inflates them and helps the physician see better.

If anything unusual is in your rectum or colon, like a polyp or inflamed tissue, the physician can remove a piece of it using instruments inserted into the scope. The physician will send that piece of tissue (biopsy) to the lab for testing.

Bleeding and puncture of the colon are possible complications of sigmoidoscopy. However, such complications are uncommon.

Sigmoidoscopy takes 10 to 20 minutes. During the procedure, you might feel pressure and slight cramping in your lower abdomen. You will feel better afterwards when the air leaves your colon.

Preparation

The colon and rectum must be completely empty for sigmoidoscopy to be thorough and safe, so the physician will probably tell you to drink only clear liquids for 12 to 24 hours beforehand. A liquid diet means fat-free bouillon or broth, Jell-O®, strained fruit juice, water, plain coffee, plain tea, or diet soda. The night before or right before the

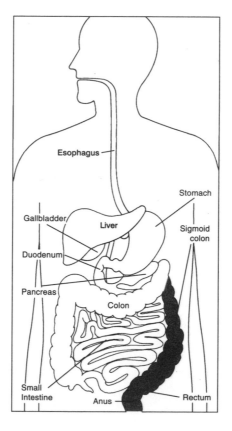

Figure 4.2. *The large intestine from the rectum through the last part of the colon is called the sigmoid colon.*

procedure, you may also be given an enema, which is a liquid solution that washes out the intestines. Your physician may give you other special instructions.

Upper Endoscopy

Upper endoscopy enables the physician to look inside the esophagus, stomach, and duodenum (first part of the small intestine). The procedure might be used to discover the reason for swallowing difficulties, nausea, vomiting, reflux, bleeding, indigestion, abdominal pain, or chest pain. Upper endoscopy is also called EGD, which stands for esophagogastroduodenoscopy.

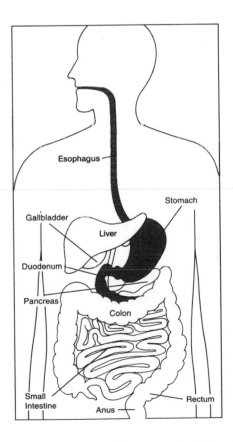

Figure 4.3. Upper endoscopy enables your physician to see inside your esophagus, stomach, and duodenum.

For the procedure you will swallow a thin, flexible, lighted tube called an endoscope. Right before the procedure the physician will spray your throat with a numbing agent that may help prevent gagging. You may also receive pain medicine and a sedative to help you relax during the exam. The endoscope transmits an image of the inside of the esophagus, stomach, and duodenum, so the physician can carefully examine the lining of these organs. The scope also blows air into the stomach; this expands the folds of tissue and makes it easier for the physician to examine the stomach.

The physician can see abnormalities, like ulcers, through the endoscope that don't show up well on x-rays. The physician can also insert instruments into the scope to remove samples of tissue (biopsy) for further tests.

Possible complications of upper endoscopy include bleeding and puncture of the stomach lining. However, such complications are rare. Most people will probably have nothing more than a mild sore throat after the procedure.

The procedure takes 20 to 30 minutes. Because you will be sedated, you will need to rest at the physician's office for 1 to 2 hours until the medication wears off.

Preparation

Your stomach and duodenum must be empty for the procedure to be thorough and safe, so you will not be able to eat or drink anything for at least 6 hours beforehand. Also, you must arrange for someone to take you home—you will not be allowed to drive because of the sedatives. Your physician may give you other special instructions.

ERCP (Endoscopic Retrograde Cholangiopancreatography)

Endoscopic retrograde cholangiopancreatography (ERCP) enables the physician to diagnose problems in the liver, gallbladder, bile ducts, and pancreas. The liver is a large organ that, among other things, makes a liquid called bile that helps with digestion. The gallbladder is a small, pear-shaped organ that stores bile until it is needed for digestion. The bile ducts are tubes that carry bile from the liver to the gallbladder and small intestine. These ducts are sometimes called the biliary tree. The pancreas is a large gland that produces chemicals that help with digestion.

ERCP may be used to discover the reason for jaundice, upper abdominal pain, and unexplained weight loss. ERCP combines the use of x-rays and an endoscope, which is a long, flexible, lighted tube. Through it, the physician can see the inside of the stomach, duodenum, and ducts in the biliary tree and pancreas.

For the procedure, you will lie on your left side on an examining table in an x-ray room. You will be given medication to help numb the back of your throat and a sedative to help you relax during the exam. You will swallow the endoscope, and the physician will then guide the scope through your esophagus, stomach, and duodenum until it reaches the spot where the ducts of the biliary tree and pancreas open into the duodenum. At this time, you will be turned to lie flat on your stomach, and the physician will pass a small plastic tube through the scope. Through the tube, the physician will inject a dye into the ducts

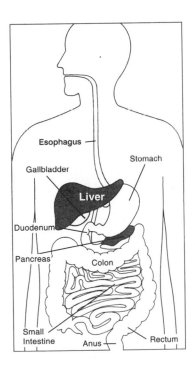

Figure 4.4. *Your physician can see inside the stomach, duodenum, and ducts in the biliary tree and pancreas using a procedure called ERCP—endoscopic retrograde cholangiopancreatography.*

to make them show up clearly on x-rays. A radiographer will begin taking x-rays as soon as the dye is injected.

If the exam shows a gallstone or narrowing of the ducts, the physician can insert instruments into the scope to remove or work around the obstruction. Also, tissue samples (biopsy) can be taken for further testing.

Possible complications of ERCP include pancreatitis (inflammation of the pancreas), infection, bleeding, and perforation of the duodenum. However, such problems are uncommon. You may have tenderness or a lump where the sedative was injected, but that should go away in a few days or weeks.

ERCP takes 30 minutes to 2 hours. You may have some discomfort when the physician blows air into the duodenum and injects the dye into the ducts. However, the pain medicine and sedative should keep you from feeling too much discomfort. After the procedure, you will need to stay at the physician's office for 1 to 2 hours until the sedative wears off. The physician will make sure you do not have signs of complications before you leave. If any kind of treatment is done during ERCP, such as removing a gallstone, you may need to stay in the hospital overnight.

Preparation

Your stomach and duodenum must be empty for the procedure to be accurate and safe. You will not be able to eat or drink anything after midnight the night before the procedure, or for 6 to 8 hours beforehand, depending on the time of your procedure. Also, the physician will need to know whether you have any allergies, especially to iodine, which is in the dye. You must also arrange for someone to take you home—you will not be allowed to drive because of the sedatives. The physician may give you other special instructions.

Lower GI Series

A lower gastrointestinal (GI) series uses x-rays to diagnose problems in the large intestine (see Figure 4.1), which includes the colon and rectum. The lower GI series may show problems like abnormal growths, ulcers, polyps, and diverticuli.

Before taking x-rays of your colon and rectum, the radiologist will put a thick liquid called barium into your colon. This is why a lower GI series is sometimes called a barium enema. The barium coats the lining of the colon and rectum and makes these organs, and any signs of disease in them, show up more clearly on x-rays. It also helps the radiologist see the size and shape of the colon and rectum.

You may be uncomfortable during the lower GI series. The barium will cause fullness and pressure in your abdomen and will make you feel the urge to have a bowel movement. However, that rarely happens because the tube the physician uses to inject the barium has a balloon on the end of it that prevents the liquid from coming back out.

You may be asked to change positions while x-rays are taken. Different positions give different views of the intestines. After the radiologist is finished taking x-rays, you will be able to go to the bathroom. The radiologist may also take an x-ray of the empty colon afterwards.

A lower GI series takes about 1 to 2 hours. The barium may cause constipation and make your stool turn gray or white for a few days after the procedure.

Preparation

Your colon must be empty for the procedure to be accurate. To prepare for the procedure you will have to restrict your diet for a few days beforehand. For example, you might be able to drink only liquids and eat only nonsugar, nondairy foods for 2 days before the procedure; only clear liquids the day before; and nothing after midnight the night before. A liquid diet means fat-free bouillon or broth, Jell-O®, strained fruit juice, water, plain coffee, plain tea, or diet soda. To make sure your colon is empty, you might be given a laxative or an enema before the procedure. Your physician may give you other special instructions.

Upper GI Series

The upper gastrointestinal (GI) series uses x-rays to diagnose problems in the esophagus, stomach, and duodenum (first part of the small intestine). It may also be used to examine the small intestine. The upper GI series can show a blockage, abnormal growth, ulcer, or a problem with the way an organ is working.

During the procedure, you will drink barium, a thick, white, milkshake-like liquid. Barium coats the inside lining of the esophagus, stomach, and duodenum and makes them show up more clearly on x-rays. The radiologist can also see ulcers, scar tissue, abnormal growths, hernias, or areas where something is blocking the normal path of food through the digestive system. Using a machine called a fluoroscope, the radiologist is also able to watch your digestive system work as the barium moves through it. This part of the procedure shows any problems in how the digestive system functions, for example, whether the muscles that control swallowing are working properly. As the barium moves into the small intestine, the radiologist can take x-rays of it as well.

An upper GI series takes 1 to 2 hours. It is not uncomfortable. The barium may cause constipation and white-colored stool for a few days after the procedure.

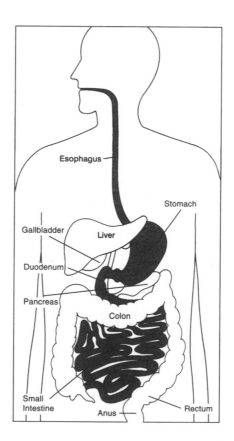

Figure 4.5. *Problems in the esophagus, stomach, duodenum, and small intestine can be diagnosed using the upper GI series.*

Preparation

Your stomach and small intestine must be empty for the procedure to be accurate, so the night before you will not be able to eat or drink anything after midnight. Your physician may give you other specific instructions.

For More Information

National Digestive Diseases Information Clearinghouse
2 Information Way
Bethesda, MD 20892-3570
Phone: (301) 654-3810
Fax: (301) 907-8906
E-mail: nddic@info.niddk.nih.gov

The National Digestive Diseases Information Clearinghouse (NDDIC) is a service of the National Institute of Diabetes and Digestive and Kidney Diseases (NIDDK). The NIDDK is part of the National Institutes of Health under the U.S. Department of Health and Human Services. Established in 1980, the clearinghouse provides information about digestive diseases to people with digestive disorders and to their families, health care professionals, and the public. NDDIC answers inquiries; develops, reviews, and distributes publications; and works closely with professional and patient organizations and Government agencies to coordinate resources about digestive diseases.

Publications produced by the clearinghouse are reviewed carefully for scientific accuracy, content, and readability.

Chapter 5

Harmful Effects of Medicines on the Adult Digestive System

Many medicines taken by mouth may affect the digestive system. These medicines include prescription (those ordered by a doctor and dispensed by a pharmacist) and nonprescription or over-the-counter (OTC) products. A glossary at the end of this chapter describes some common prescription and nonprescription medicines discussed below that may affect the digestive system.

Although these medicines usually are safe and effective, harmful effects may occur in some people. OTC's typically do not cause serious side effects when taken as directed on the product's label. It is important to read the label to find out the ingredients, side effects, warnings, and when to consult a doctor.

Always talk with your doctor before taking a medicine for the first time and before adding any new medicines to those you already are taking. Tell the doctor about all other medicines (prescription and OTC's) you are taking. Certain medicines taken together may interact and cause harmful side effects. In addition, tell the doctor about any allergies or sensitivities to foods and medicines and about any medical conditions you may have such as diabetes, kidney disease, or liver disease.

National Institute of Diabetes and Digestive and Kidney Diseases (NIDDK), NIH Publication No. 95-3421, September 1992. The U.S. Government does not endorse or favor any specific commercial product or company. Brand names appearing in this publication are used only because they are considered essential in the context of the information reported herein.

Be sure that you understand all directions for taking the medicine, including dose and schedule, possible interactions with food, alcohol, and other medicines, side effects, and warnings. If you are an older adult read all directions carefully and ask your doctor questions about the medicine. As you get older, you may be more susceptible to drug interactions that cause side effects.

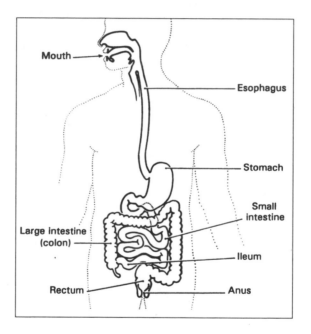

Figure 5.1.

People with a food intolerance such as gluten intolerance should make sure their medicines do not contain fillers or additives with gluten.

Check with your doctor if you have any questions or concerns about your medicines. Follow the doctor's orders carefully, and immediately report any unusual symptoms or the warning signs described below.

The Esophagus

Irritation

Some people have difficulty swallowing medicines in tablet or capsule form. Tablets or capsules that stay in the esophagus may release chemicals that irritate the lining of the esophagus. The irritation may cause ulcers, bleeding, perforation (a hole or tear), and strictures (narrowing) of the esophagus. The risk of pill-induced injuries to the esophagus increases in persons with conditions involving the esophagus, such as strictures, scleroderma (hardening of the skin), achalasia (irregular muscle activity of the esophagus, which delays the passage of food), and stroke.

Some medicines can cause ulcers when they become lodged in the esophagus. These medicines include aspirin, several antibiotics such as tetracycline, quinidine, potassium chloride, vitamin C, and iron.

Warning Signs

- Pain when swallowing food or liquid.
- Feeling of a tablet or capsule "stuck" in the throat.
- Dull, aching pain in the chest or shoulder after taking medicines.

Precautions

- Swallow tablets or capsules while you are in an upright or sitting position.

- Before taking a tablet or capsule, swallow several sips of liquid to lubricate the throat, then swallow the tablet or capsule with at least a full glass (8 ounces) of liquid.

- Do not lie down immediately after taking medicines to ensure that the pills pass through the esophagus into the stomach.

- Tell your doctor if painful swallowing continues or if pills continue to stick in the throat.

Esophageal Reflux

The lower esophageal sphincter (LES) muscle is between the esophagus and the stomach. The muscle allows the passage of food into the stomach after swallowing. Certain medicines interfere with the action of the sphincter muscle, which increases the likelihood of backup or reflux of the highly acidic contents of the stomach into the esophagus.

Medicines that can cause esophageal reflux include nitrates, theophylline, calcium channel blockers, anticholinergics, and birth control pills.

Warning Signs

- Heartburn or indigestion.
- Sensation of food coming back up into the throat.

Precautions

- Avoid foods and beverages that may worsen reflux, including coffee, alcohol, chocolate, and fried or fatty foods.
- Cut down on, or preferably quit, smoking.
- Do not lie down immediately after eating.

The Stomach

Irritation

One of the most common drug-induced injuries is irritation of the lining of the stomach caused by nonsteroidal anti-inflammatory drugs (NSAIDs).

NSAIDs can irritate the stomach by weakening the ability of the lining to resist acid made in the stomach. Sometimes this irritation may lead to inflammation of the stomach lining (gastritis), ulcers, bleeding, or perforation of the lining.

In addition, you should be aware that stomach irritation may occur without having any of the symptoms below.

Older people are especially at risk for irritation from NSAIDs because they are more likely to regularly take pain medicines for arthritis and other chronic conditions. Also at risk are individuals with a history of peptic ulcers and related complications or gastritis. These individuals should tell their doctor about any of these previous conditions. Special medicines may be needed to protect the stomach lining.

Warning Signs

- Severe stomach cramps or pain or burning in the stomach or back.

- Black, tarry, or bloody stools.
- Bloody vomit.
- Severe heartburn or indigestion.
- Diarrhea.

Precautions

- Use coated tablets, which may lessen stomach irritation.
- Avoid drinking alcoholic beverages while taking medicines.
- Take medicines with a full glass of water or milk or with food, which may reduce irritation.

Delayed Emptying of the Stomach

Some medicines cause nerve and muscle activity to slow down in the stomach. This slowing down causes the contents of the stomach to empty at a slower rate than normal.

Drugs that may cause this delay include anticholinergics and drugs used to treat Parkinson's disease and depression.

Warning Signs

- Nausea.
- Bloating.
- Feeling of fullness.
- Vomiting of food eaten many hours earlier.
- Pain in mid-abdomen.
- Heartburn or indigestion.
- Sensation of food coming back up into the throat.

Precautions

- Eat frequent, small meals.
- Do not lie down for about 30 minutes after eating.
- Tell your doctor if symptoms continue. Your doctor may consider changing your dosage of the medicine or trying a new medicine.

The Intestine

Constipation

Constipation can be caused by a variety of medicines. These medicines affect the nerve and muscle activity in the large intestine (colon).

This results in the slow and difficult passage of stool. Medicines also may bind intestinal liquid and make the stool hard.

Medicines that commonly cause constipation include antihypertensives, anticholinergics, cholestyramine, iron, and antacids that contain mostly aluminium.

Warning Sign

- Constipation that is severe or disabling or that lasts several weeks.

Precautions

- Drink plenty of fluids.
- Eat a well-balanced diet that includes whole grains, fruits, and vegetables.
- Exercise regularly.
- Take laxatives only under a doctor's supervision.

Diarrhea

Diarrhea is a common side effect of many medicines. Diarrhea is often caused by antibiotics, which affect the bacteria that live normally in the large intestine.

Antibiotic-induced changes in intestinal bacteria allow overgrowth of another bacteria, *Clostridium difficile* (*C. difficile*), which is the cause of a more serious antibiotic-induced diarrhea.

The presence of *C. difficile* can cause colitis, an inflammation of the intestine in which the bowel "weeps" excess water and mucus, resulting in loose, watery stools. Almost any antibiotic may cause *C. difficile*-induced diarrhea, but the most common are ampicillin, clindamycin, and the cephalosporins. Antibiotic-induced colitis is treated with another antibiotic that acts on *C. difficile*.

Diarrhea also can be a side effect of drugs that do not cause colitis but that alter the movements or fluid content of the colon. Colchicine is a common cause of drug-induced diarrhea. Magnesium-containing antacids can have the effect of laxatives and cause diarrhea if overused. In addition, the abuse of laxatives may result in damage to the nerves and muscles of the colon and cause diarrhea.

Warning Signs

- Blood, mucus, or pus in the stool.

- Pain in the lower abdomen.
- Fever.

Precaution

- If diarrhea lasts for several days, consult your doctor.

The Liver

The liver processes most medicines that enter the bloodstream and governs drug activity throughout the body. Once a drug enters the bloodstream, the liver converts the drug into chemicals the body can use and removes toxic chemicals that other organs cannot tolerate. During this process, these chemicals can attack and injure the liver.

Drug-induced liver injury can resemble the symptoms of any acute or chronic liver disease. The only way a doctor can diagnose drug-induced liver injury is by stopping use of the suspected drug and excluding other liver diseases through diagnostic tests. Rarely, long-term use of a medicine can cause chronic liver damage and scarring (cirrhosis).

Medicines that can cause severe liver injury include large doses of acetaminophen (and even in small doses when taken with alcohol), anticonvulsants such as phenytoin and valproic acid, the antihypertensive methyldopa, the tranquilizer chlorpromazine, antituberculins used to treat tuberculosis such as isoniazid and rifampin, and vitamins such as vitamin A and niacin.

Warning Signs (for liver injury)

- Severe fatigue.
- Abdominal pain and swelling.
- Jaundice (yellow eyes and skin, dark urine).
- Fever.
- Nausea or vomiting.

Precautions

- If you have ever had a liver disease or gallstones, you should discuss this with your doctor before taking any medicines that may affect the liver or the gallbladder.

- Take these medicines only in the prescribed or recommended doses.

43

Glossary of Medicines

The following glossary is a guide to medicines used to treat many medical conditions. The glossary does not include all medicines that may affect the digestive system. If a medicine you are taking is not listed here, check with your doctor.

Acetaminophen. Acetaminophen relieves fever and pain by blocking pain centers in the central nervous system. Examples of brand names include Tylenol, Panadol, and Datril.

Antacids. Antacids relieve heartburn, acid indigestion, sour stomach, and symptoms of peptic ulcer. They work by neutralizing stomach acid. Aluminum hydroxide antacids include Alu-Tab and Amphojel; calcium carbonate antacids include Tums, Alka Mints, and Rolaids Calcium Rich; magnesium antacids include Mylanta and Maalox.

Antibiotics. Antibiotics destroy or block the growth of bacteria that cause infection. Hundreds of antibiotics are available, including penicillins (Amoxil, Amcil, and Augmentin), clindamycin, cephalosporins (Keflex and Ceclor), tetracyclines (Minocin, Sumycin, and Vibramycin), quinolones (Cipro), and sulfa drugs (Bactrim).

Anticholinergics. This class of medicines affects the nerve cells or nerve fibers and includes drugs for depression, anxiety, and nervousness. Examples of anticholinergics include propantheline (Probanthine) and dicyclomine (Bentyl). Examples of antidepressants include amitriptyline (Elavil and Endep), and nortriptyline (Aventyl and Pamelor).

Medicines for relieving the symptoms of Parkinson's disease also are in this category. Examples include levodopa (Dopar) and carbidopa and levodopa combination (Sinemet).

Anticonvulsants. These medicines control epilepsy and other types of seizure disorders. They act by lessening overactive nerve impulses in the brain. Examples of this class of medicines include phenytoin (Dilantin) and valproic acid (Dalpro).

Antihypertensives. Antihypertensives lower high blood pressure. They act by relaxing blood vessels, which makes blood flow more easily. Examples of antihypertensives include methyldopa (Aldomet) and clonidine hydrochloride (Catapres).

Antituberculins. These drugs for tuberculosis limit the growth of bacteria or prevent tuberculosis from developing in people who have a positive tuberculin skin test. Brand names include INH, Dow-Isoniazid, Rifadin, and Rimactane.

Calcium channel blockers. These medicines for angina (chest pain) and high blood pressure affect the movement of calcium into the cells of the heart and blood vessels, relax blood vessels, and increase the flow of blood and oxygen to the heart. Examples of calcium channel blockers include diltiazem (Cardizem), nifedipine (Procardia), and verpamil (Isoptin).

Chlorpromazine. This tranquilizer relieves anxiety or agitation. Examples of brand names include Thorazine and Ormazine.

Colchicine. This medicine eases the inflammation from gout and prevents attacks from recurring.

Iron. Iron is a mineral the body needs to produce red blood cells. Iron supplements are used to treat iron deficiency or iron-deficiency anemia.

Laxatives. Many forms of laxatives are available for relieving constipation. Common brand names of laxatives include Phillips' Milk of Magnesia, Citroma, Epsom salts, Correctol, and ExLax.

Nitrates. These drugs for angina (chest pain) relax blood vessels and increase the flow of blood to the heart. Examples of generic and brand names include isosorbide dinitrate (Iso-Bid and Isonate) and nitroglycerin (Nitro-Bid and Nitrocap).

Nonsteroidal anti-inflammatory drugs (NSAIDs). These drugs block the body's production of prostaglandins, substances that mediate pain and inflammation. NSAIDs relieve the pain from chronic and acute inflammatory conditions, including arthritis and other rheumatic conditions, and pain associated with injuries, bursitis, tendinitis, and dental problems. NSAIDs also relieve pain associated with noninflammatory conditions. Generic and brand names of NSAIDs include aspirin (Bayer and Bufferin), ibuprofen (Advil, Nuprin, and Motrin), tometin (Tolectin), naproxen (Naprosyn), and piroxicam (Feldene).

Potassium chloride. Potassium is a vital element in the body. Potassium supplements help prevent and treat potassium deficiency in people taking diuretics.

Quinidine. This medicine often is used to correct irregular heartbeat. Brand names of quinidine include Quinalan and Quiniglute.

Theophylline. This medicine eases breathing difficulties associated with emphysema, bronchitis, and bronchial asthma. The medicine works by relaxing the muscles of the respiratory tract, which allows an easier flow of air into the lungs. Examples of brand names include Theo-Dur, Theophyl, and Bronkodyl.

Vitamins. Vitamins serve as nutritional supplements in people with poor diets, in people recovering from surgery, or in people with special health problems.

- Niacin helps the body break down food for energy and is used to treat niacin deficiency and to lower levels of fats and cholesterol.

- Vitamin A is necessary for normal growth and for healthy eyes and skin.

- Vitamin C is necessary for healthy function of cells.

Additional Readings

AARP Pharmacy Service Prescription Drug Handbook. Glenview, Illinois: Scott, Foreman and Company, 1988. General reference book for the public by the American Association of Retired Persons that provides information about medicines most frequently prescribed for persons over 50 years of age.

Advice for the Patient: Drug Information in Lay Language, USP DI, 12th edition. Rockville, Maryland: The United States Pharmacopeial Convention, 1992. Guide for the patient that provides information about medicines by brand and generic names in sections on dosage forms, proper use directions, precautions, and side effects.

Drug Information for the Health Care Professional, USP DI, 12th edition. Rockville, Maryland: The United States Pharmacopeial Convention, 1992. Guide for health care professionals that provides information about medicines by brand and generic names in sections on pharmacology, indications, precautions, side effects, general dosing, dosage forms, and patient consultation.

Kimmey, MG. Gastroduodenal effects of nonsteroidal anti-inflammatory drugs. *Postgraduate Medicine*, 1989; 85(5): 65-71. General review article for primary care physicians.

Physicians' Desk Reference, 46th edition. Montvale, New Jersey: Medical Economics Company, Inc., 1992. Reference book for health care professionals that includes information about 2,800 pharmaceutical products in sections on pharmacology, indications, contraindications, precautions, adverse reactions, and dosage and administration.

Stehlin, D. How to take your medicine: nonsteroidal anti-inflammatory drugs. *FDA Consumer*, 1990; 24(5): 33-35. General review article for the public.

Additional Resources

National Council on Patient Information and Education
666 11th Street NW., Suite 810
Washington, DC 20001
(202) 347-6711

Distributes resources to the public and health care professionals about prescription medicines.

The United States Pharmacopeial Convention, Inc.
12601 Twinbrook Parkway
Rockville, MD 20852
(301) 881-0666

Distributes information about drug use and drug standards to health professionals and the public.

National Digestive Diseases Information Clearinghouse
2 Information Way
Bethesda, MD 20892-3570
E-mail: nddic@info.niddk.nih.gov

The National Digestive Diseases Information Clearinghouse (NDDIC) is a service of the National Institute of Diabetes and Digestive and Kidney Diseases (NIDDK). The NIDDK is part of the National Institutes of Health under the U.S. Public Health Service. Established in 1980, the clearinghouse provides information about digestive diseases to people with digestive disorders and to their families, health care professionals, and the public. NDDIC answers inquiries; develops, reviews, and distributes publications; and works closely with professional and patient organizations and Government agencies to coordinate resources about digestive diseases.

Publications produced by the clearinghouse are reviewed carefully for scientific accuracy, content, and readability.

Chapter 6

Smoking and Your Digestive System

Introduction

Cigarette smoking causes a variety of life-threatening diseases, including lung cancer, emphysema, and heart disease. An estimated 400,000 deaths each year are caused directly by cigarette smoking. Smoking is responsible for changes in all parts of the body, including the digestive system. This fact can have serious consequences because it is the digestive system that converts foods into the nutrients the body needs to live.

Current estimates indicate that about one-third of all adults smoke. And, while adult men seem to be smoking less, women and teenagers of both sexes seem to be smoking more. How does smoking affect the digestive system of all these people?

Questions and Answers about Smoking and Your Digestive System

What Are Some of the Harmful Effects of Smoking on the Digestive System?

Smoking has been shown to have harmful effects on all parts of the digestive system, contributing to such common disorders as heartburn and peptic ulcers. The effects of smoking on the liver often are

National Institute of Diabetes and Digestive and Kidney Diseases (NIDDK), National Institute of Health, NIH Pub. No. 95-949, 1995.

not discussed, but studies show that smoking may alter the way in which the liver handles drugs and alcohol. In addition, smoking apparently changes the way in which food is processed by the body. In fact, there seems to be enough evidence to stop smoking solely on the basis of digestive distress.

How Does Smoking Contribute to Heartburn?

Heartburn is a very common disorder among Americans. Heartburn is especially common among pregnant women, with 25 percent reporting daily heartburn and more than 50 percent experiencing occasional distress.

Most people will experience heartburn if the lining of the esophagus comes into contact with too much stomach juice for a long period of time. This stomach juice consists of acid produced by the stomach, as well as bile salts and digestive enzymes that may have washed into the stomach from the intestine.

Normally, a muscular valve at the lower end of the esophagus, the lower esophageal sphincter (LES), keeps the acid solution in the stomach and out of the esophagus. Sometimes the LES is weak and allows stomach juice to reflux, or flow backward into the esophagus.

Many people have occasional reflux episodes. Persons with heartburn usually have frequent episodes or fail to return the refluxed material to the stomach promptly. The prolonged contact of acid stomach juice with the esophageal lining injures the esophagus and produces burning pain. Smoking decreases the strength of the esophageal valve, thereby allowing more refluxed material into the esophagus.

Smoking also seems to promote the movement of bile salts from the intestine to the stomach to produce a more harmful reflux material. Finally, smoking may directly injure the esophagus, making it less able to resist further damage because of contact with refluxed material from the stomach.

Does Smoking Cause Peptic Ulcers?

An ulcer is an open sore in the lining of the stomach or duodenum, the first part of the small intestine. The exact cause of ulcers is not known. A relationship between smoking cigarettes and ulcers, especially duodenal ulcers, does exist. The 1989 Surgeon General's report stated that ulcers are more likely to occur, less likely to heal, and more likely to cause death in smokers than in nonsmokers.

Why is this so? Doctors are not really sure, but smoking does seem to be one of several factors that work together to promote the formation of ulcers.

Stomach acid is important in producing ulcers. Normally, most of this acid is buffered by the food we eat. Most of the unbuffered acid that enters the duodenum is quickly neutralized by sodium bicarbonate, a naturally occurring alkali produced by the pancreas. Some studies show that smoking reduces the bicarbonate produced by the pancreas, interfering with the neutralization of acid in the duodenum. Other studies suggest that chronic cigarette smoking may increase the amount of acid secreted by the stomach.

There also is some evidence suggesting that smoking increases the speed at which the stomach empties its acid contents into the small intestine. Although the evidence is inconclusive on some of these issues, all are possible explanations for the higher rate and slower healing of ulcers among smokers.

Whatever causes the link between smoking and ulcers, two points have been repeatedly demonstrated: Persons who smoke are more likely to develop an ulcer, especially a duodenal ulcer, and ulcers are less likely to heal quickly among smokers in response to otherwise effective treatment. This research tracing the relationship between smoking and ulcers strongly suggests that a person with an ulcer should stop smoking.

How Does Smoking Affect the Liver?

The liver is a very important organ that has many tasks. Among other things, the liver is responsible for processing drugs, alcohol, and other toxins to remove them from the body. There is evidence that smoking alters the ability of the liver to handle these substances. In some cases, this may influence the dose of medication necessary to treat an illness. One theory, based on current evidence also suggests that smoking can aggravate the course of liver disease caused by excessive alcohol intake.

Does Smoking Help Control Weight?

A common belief is that smoking helps to control weight. Smokers do, indeed, weigh less, on the average, than nonsmokers. And those who quit smoking are more likely to gain weight. Most people think this is because smokers eat less than nonsmokers.

Some researchers have found, however, that smokers actually eat more than nonsmokers. How can they weigh less? What happens to the extra calories? Scientists are not really sure about the answers to these questions, but they caution smokers not to think that just because they weigh less, they are healthier than if they didn't smoke. Research shows that the bodies of smokers use food less efficiently than nonsmokers. Scientists are still studying what implications this has on the long-range health of smokers.

Can the Damage to the Digestive System Be Reversed?

Some of the effects of smoking on the digestive system appear to be of short duration. For example, the effect of smoking on bicarbonate production by the pancreas does not appear to last. Within a half-hour after smoking, the production of bicarbonate returns to normal. The effects of smoking on how the liver handles drugs also disappear when a person stops smoking. While doctors suspect that most other digestive abnormalities caused by smoking would also disappear soon after stopping smoking, this question has received little study.

Summary

While all the evidence is not yet available, it seems clear that smoking cigarettes plays an important role in causing some digestive diseases. The relationship between heartburn and smoking is very clear. The link between smoking and ulcers, especially duodenal ulcers, seems indisputable. Studies showing that cigarettes affect the way the liver processes drugs, alcohol, and other substances suggest more problems for smokers.

Not all the effects of smoking on the digestive system are understood clearly. However, the evidence that is available makes a powerful statement that smoking is bad for digestive health.

Additional Readings

National Digestive Diseases Information Clearinghouse. Provides information about digestive diseases, including heartburn and peptic ulcer. 2 Information Way, Bethesda, MD 20892-3570.

Office on Smoking and Health, Public Information Branch. Publishes and distributes materials on smoking and health, including the Surgeon General's annual reports. 4770 Buford Highway NE., Mail Stop K50, Atlanta, GA 30341-3724; (404) 488-5705.

Chapter 7

When Do You Need an Antacid?

You can't believe you ate the whole thing. But you did. All seven courses. Then you had two helpings of dessert. Then, to be social, you had a couple of drinks. Or maybe three or four.

And now you're paying for it. You've got a "burning sensation" in your stomach or your chest, or maybe you feel all knotted up inside.

Your first reaction may be to reach for your favorite antacid to make the hurting go away. And if you do, you won't be alone.

Americans are currently spending close to $1 billion per year on these popular, over-the-counter drugs. Used according to directions and in moderation, they can quickly relieve the symptoms associated with occasional heartburn and indigestion. But these useful products may not always be necessary, and they have their dark side if used improperly.

"Improperly" means taking too much of an antacid over a short period, or using antacids frequently over a long period (weeks, months or years). Frequent and prolonged use of these products can cause irreparable harm to your heart, kidneys or bones.

Even if used occasionally and in moderation, antacids can mean bad news for people with special medical conditions.

Hugo Gallo-Torres, M.D., a medical officer with FDA's Center for Drug Evaluation and Research, said it's a good idea to consult your doctor before using antacids if you:

"A Burning Question: When Do You Need an Antacid?" by Tom Cramer, *FDA Consumer*, January/February 1992.

- are on any kind of medication
- are pregnant or breast-feeding
- have kidney problems
- have chronic constipation, diarrhea or colitis
- have stomach or intestinal bleeding
- have an irregular heartbeat
- have any kind of chronic illness
- have symptoms that may indicate appendicitis

Though they cause problems for some, most people can take antacids without worrying. Consumers who use them only once in a while, and as directed, are unlikely to experience significant side effects.

But, like most everything else in life, moderation is the key.

"Antacids are useful drugs—they serve a purpose," said Gallo-Torres. "Ideally, though, it's always better to try dealing with heartburn and indigestion—at least initially—without taking any medications at all, or by avoiding trouble in the first place."

Gallo-Torres said there are some simple steps you can take that may help prevent heartburn or indigestion.

- Don't eat big meals. Your stomach has to work long and hard to process them, which means it has to produce a lot of acid. It helps to eat more frequent—but smaller—meals.

- Eat more slowly. Downing a lot of food in a hurry can overwhelm your stomach, which responds by producing extra digestive acids.

- After you eat, don't lie down right away. If you do, you're more likely to have heartburn, because gravity is now preventing food from going speedily to the intestines. It's also a good idea to eat your last big meal at least three hours before bedtime. When you go to sleep, everything slows down, including your digestive system, so food you've eaten right before bedtime will stay in your stomach longer. It won't feel good.

- Don't wear tight-fitting garments. They can literally compress your stomach, making it more likely that the stomach's acid contents will enter your esophagus and cause a burning sensation.

- Cut down on caffeine; it makes your stomach produce more acid. Caffeine-heavy items include coffee, tea, chocolate, and some sodas.

- Avoid foods that contain a lot of acid, such as citrus fruits and tomatoes, and any other food that gives you problems.

- Cut back on alcohol and smoking. Both irritate the lining of your stomach and both tend to lower esophageal sphincter pressure. When this happens, it's easier for the contents of your stomach to shoot back up into your esophagus.

- Sleep with your head and shoulders propped up six to eight inches, so that your body is at a slight angle. This gets gravity working for you and not against you, and the digestive juices in your stomach are more likely to head south, for your intestine, instead of back up into your esophagus.

"If you do take an antacid, remember that what you're taking is a drug," Gallo-Torres said. "It is a drug that, in the vast majority of cases, should be used only for occasional relief of mild heartburn or indigestion. Antacids are fast-acting. They should bring relief within minutes. If you're taking antacids and there's no relief, then something else may be going on, something that requires a physician's evaluation."

Igor Cerny, a pharmacist with FDA's Center for Drug Evaluation and Research, agreed. "If you find yourself taking antacids frequently," he said, "you need to say to yourself: 'Wait a minute.... I wasn't doing this before, so why am I doing it now? Something might be wrong with me.'"

"If your symptoms last more than two weeks, go see your doctor," he recommended. "Two weeks is the general rule of thumb. Beyond that, taking antacids can actually mask a more serious medical problem."

Cerny said it's a good idea to see your doctor even sooner—preferably right away—if you're experiencing any symptoms severe enough to interfere with our lifestyle, symptoms such as continuous vomiting or diarrhea, extreme discomfort or pain in your gastrointestinal (GI) tract, vomiting of blood or material that looks like coffee grounds (but which is actually digested blood), or any of these accompanied by fever.

"Using antacids to alleviate serious symptoms like these is like trying to put out a building fire with a hand-held extinguisher," Cerny said. "Serious symptoms require professional evaluation and treatment."

A Quick Look Inside

Your entire digestive system is called the alimentary canal, or GI tract. About 30 feet from beginning to end, it includes your mouth (where digestion actually begins), esophagus, stomach, small intestine, and colon (also called the large intestine). Antacids do most of their work in the stomach.

The stomach serves as a kind of "holding tank" for food before it moves on to the intestines, where the major part of digestion takes place. But the stomach does more than just hold food. It helps with digestion, too. It secretes pepsin and hydrochloric acid, which work together to break down proteins into simpler compounds.

Under normal conditions, the digestive process rolls along quietly and efficiently, unnoticed. But every once in a while something happens down there that catches your attention: a burning sensation, a cramped or bloated feeling, or other unpleasant phenomena that tell you something is not quite right.

The pH Factor

Antacids make you feel better by increasing the pH balance in your stomach. The pH system is a scale for measuring the acidity or alkalinity of a given environment (in this case, your stomach). The scale goes from zero to 14.

Seven is neutral. Below seven is acid. Above seven is alkaline.

Normally, the acid level in your stomach is about 2 or 3. Trouble may start when your pH drops below those numbers.

To make you feel better, an antacid need not bring the pH level all the way up to 7 (neutral), which would be a highly unnatural state for your stomach anyway. In order to work, all the antacid has to do is get you to 3 or 4. It does this by neutralizing some of the excess acid.

So What's Wrong with Me Anyway?

The world of gastrointestinal disorders is a complex and sometimes baffling one. If you're feeling pain or discomfort in your GI tract, it could be something as unworrisome as simple indigestion, or maybe a stress ulcer.

Or it could be cancer.

In between these extremes are a billion other possibilities (a slight exaggeration, but you get the idea).

For example, your doctor may say you're suffering from non-ulcer dyspepsia. According to the *Handbook of Nonprescription Drugs* (ninth edition), non-ulcer dyspepsia "refers to intermittent [on and off] upper abdominal discomfort, the cause of which is not clearly defined."

In other words, when you get right down to it, non-ulcer dyspepsia is a catch-all term used for all sorts of stomach upset problems.

Some symptoms include upper abdominal pain, nausea, vomiting, bloating, and indigestion.

Indigestion is another fuzzy word. Some people like to call it sour stomach, or acid indigestion, or upset stomach, or acid stomach.

It could mean that you have a touch of gastritis (when your stomach lining becomes inflamed by too much acid secretion). Or it could mean you've simply eaten too much at once, and all that food is sitting heavy in your stomach, like a bowling ball, trying to get digested (as in the case of the massive overindulgence described at the beginning of this article).

Then there's heartburn, which is another matter.

Heartburn happens when the stomach's contents, along with all its corrosive digestive juices, goes into reverse and shoots back up into the esophagus (the tube that extends from the pharynx, or throat, into the stomach). Normally, the pressure in your stomach is lower than the pressure in your esophagus, which helps prevent food from reentering the esophagus. But once in a while the delicate pressure system can break down.

This unsettling event, called gastroesophageal reflux (heartburn), may sometimes announce itself with an embarrassing belch.

But whether you make a noise or not, you feel the burning. The lining of your stomach is fairly accustomed to an acid environment, but your esophagus definitely isn't, so even a little acid in there will sometimes be enough to get your attention.

If gastroesophageal reflux is happening to you all the time, then you may have something called gastroesophageal reflux disease. It could be that your esophageal sphincter (the "door" between your esophagus and your stomach) is weak, chronically allowing the stomach's contents to push back out into the esophagus, burning it.

If the burning sensation is a little lower, and stays around for more than a few days, you could have another problem altogether: a peptic ulcer. An ulcer is simply a sore in your stomach that keeps getting irritated by all the acid swirling around down there.

Antacids can be used to treat all these GI problems. But most people who experience occasional discomfort somewhere along the GI tract, are likely not dealing with an ulcer, or stomach cancer, or anything else major.

Chances are it's run-of-the-mill heartburn or indigestion.

You don't need to see a doctor for occasional heartburn or indigestion. The hurting will disappear on its own. If you want some relief in the meantime, antacids will fit the bill nicely.

Again, it should be emphasized that if you experience unpleasant GI symptoms for more than two weeks, or if your symptoms are severe, it may be more than something run-of-the-mill.

Get it checked out.

Recipe for Relief

FDA requires that every antacid on the market be safe (which means the antacid won't cause serious side effects, provided you take it in the proper dosage over the recommended period of time) and effective (which means the antacid will do what it's supposed to do).

Drug manufacturers must make and label their antacids according to specific guidelines in FDA's monograph on antacids. If manufacturers don't follow this federal antacids "recipe," they are not allowed to market their products.

According to FDA's monograph, an antacid is safe and effective if it meets the following conditions:

- It must contain at least one of the antacid active ingredients (acid neutralizers) approved by the agency. (All the approved ingredients are listed in the antacid monograph.)

- It must contain a sufficient amount of the active ingredients. Specifically, each active ingredient included in the antacid product must contribute at least 25 percent to the product's total neutralizing capacity.

- In a laboratory test, the antacid must neutralize a specific amount of acid and keep it neutralized for at least 10 minutes.

- The label on the antacid must state that the product is good only for relieving the symptoms of "heartburn," "sour stomach," "acid indigestion," and "upset stomach associated with these symptoms." The label can't make any other medical claims.

- The label must contain certain warnings concerning proper dosage, side effects (such as constipation or diarrhea), and how much sodium the product contains.

- The label must warn about the product's possible interactions with other drugs. Antacids can increase or decrease the speed at which some medications are eliminated from the body. For example, antacids can block the body's absorption of tetracycline, an antibiotic.

- The label must give directions for using the product, and it must carry a warning not to use the product for more than two weeks except under the advice and supervision of a physician.

What's in an Antacid?

The opposite of an acid is a base, and that's exactly what antacids are.

But a base all by itself can't neutralize the acid inside you. For reasons that are best explained on a blackboard in chemistry class, a base needs some chemical "helpers," or ingredients, to accompany it on its neutralizing mission into your stomach.

All antacids contain at least one of the four primary "helpers" or ingredients: sodium, calcium, magnesium, and aluminum.

Here's a brief rundown of the composition and some potential side effects of various antacids:

Sodium (Alka-Seltzer, Bromo Seltzer, and Others)

Sodium bicarbonate or baking soda, perhaps the best known of the sodium-containing antacids, is potent and fast-acting. As its name suggests, it's heavy in sodium. If you're on a salt-restricted diet, and especially if the diet is intended to treat high blood pressure, take a sodium-containing antacid only under a doctor's orders.

Calcium (Tums, Alka-2, Titralac, and Others)

Antacids in the form of calcium carbonate or calcium phosphate are potent and fast-acting.

Regular or heavy doses of calcium (more than five or six times per week) can cause constipation. Heavy and extended use of this product may clog your kidneys and cut down the amount of blood they can process, and can also cause kidney stones.

Magnesium (Maalox, Mylanta, Camalox, Riopan, Gelusil, and Others)

Magnesium salts come in many forms—carbonate, glycinate, hydroxide, oxide, trisilicate, and aluminosilicates. Magnesium has a mild laxative effect; it can cause diarrhea. For this reason, magnesium salts are rarely used as the only active ingredients in an antacid, but are combined with aluminum, which counteracts the laxative effect. (The brand names listed above all contain magnesium-aluminum combinations.)

Like calcium, magnesium may cause kidney stones if taken for a very prolonged period, especially if the kidneys are functioning improperly to begin with. A serious magnesium overload in the bloodstream (hypermagnesemia) can also cause blood pressure to drop, leading to respiratory or cardiac depression—a potentially dangerous decrease in lung or heart function.

Aluminum (Rolaids, ALternaGEL, Amphogel, and Others)

Salts of aluminum (hydroxide, carbonate gel, or phosphate gel) can also cause constipation. For these reasons, aluminum is usually used in combination with the other three primary ingredients.

Used heavily over an extended period, antacids containing aluminum can weaken bones—especially in people who have kidney problems. Aluminum can cause dietary phosphates, calcium and fluoride to leave the body, eventually causing bone problems such as osteomalacia or osteoporosis.

It should be emphasized that aluminum-containing antacids present virtually no danger to people with normal kidney function who use these products only occasionally and as directed.

Simethicone

Some antacids contain an ingredient called simethicone, a gastric defoaming agent that breaks up gas bubbles, making them easier to eliminate from your body.

FDA says simethicone is safe and effective in combination with antacids for relief of gas associated with heartburn. But not all antacids contain this ingredient.

If you're looking for relief of symptoms associated with gas, read the antacid's label carefully to make sure it contains simethicone.

—by Tom Cramer

Tom Cramer is a staff writer for FDA Consumer.

Chapter 8

Remedies for Upset Stomachs

A vague queasiness stirs in your stomach. Queasy quickly turns to severely nauseated. A sour bubble rises in your throat, and you dash for the bathroom in a cold sweat.

Whatever the cause, the nausea and vomiting of an upset stomach are nasty. Upset stomachs caused by motion or too much food or drink may respond to over-the-counter (OTC) medicines. For other upset stomachs, professional care and no medication often are best.

Motion Sickness

Paleness, yawning and restlessness often precede the nausea, vomiting and dizziness that occur in motion sickness, which most frequently strikes youngsters ages 2 to 12, but may occur at any age.

The primary culprit in this condition is excess stimulation to the inner ear's maze of fluid-filled canals, responsible for maintaining the body's balance. Poor ventilation, anxiety or other emotional upset, and visual stimuli may contribute to motion sickness.

Because motion sickness is easier to prevent than to treat once it has begun, it may help to take an OTC drug to prevent symptoms 30 to 60 minutes before traveling and then continue doses during travel.

This chapter contains text from "Taming Tummy Turmoil," by Dixie Farley, *FDA Consumer*, June 1996 with revisions made in November 1996, Pub. No. (FDA) 96-3219; and "OTC Drugs for Upset Stomachs," an undated fact sheet produced by the U.S. Food and Drug Administration.

The Food and Drug Administration considers four active ingredients to be safe and effective for use in OTC drugs for motion sickness, says Gerald Rachanow, deputy director of the monograph review staff in FDA's Office of OTC Drug Evaluation. The ingredients are cyclizine (Marezine and others), dimenhydrinate (Dramamine and others), diphenhydramine (Benadryl and others), and meclizine (Bonine and others).

The active ingredients in these drugs are antihistamines. Their main side effect is drowsiness. Alcohol, tranquilizers and sedatives may increase this effect. Rachanow says anyone taking a drug for motion sickness should use caution when driving a vehicle or operating machinery and should avoid alcoholic beverages.

In large doses, OTC drugs for motion sickness may cause dry mouth and, rarely, blurred vision. "People with breathing problems such as emphysema or chronic bronchitis, glaucoma, or urinating difficulty due to an enlarged prostate should not take these drugs unless directed to do so by a doctor," Rachanow says.

OTC drugs for motion sickness have the following age restrictions:

- cyclizine—not for use under age 6
- dimenhydrinate—not for use under age 2
- diphenhydramine—not for use under age 6
- meclizine—not for use under age 12.

Before trying these drugs, or along with them, the following measures may also help stave off motion sickness:

- Don't read during travel.
- Keep your line of vision fairly straight ahead.
- Avoid excess food or alcohol before and during extended travel.
- Avoid all food and drinks on short trips.
- Stay where motion is felt the least—the front seat of a car, near the wings of an airplane, or amidship (preferably on deck).
- Avoid tobacco smoke and other odors, particularly from food.

Heartburn

FDA recently approved four drugs for OTC use that work systemically to reduce the amount of stomach acid produced. They are also sold by prescription at higher dosage levels to treat gastrointestinal illnesses such as ulcers.

Pepcid AC Acid Controller (famotidine), Tagamet HB (cimetidine), and Axid AR (nizatidine) are marketed OTC as a preventative before consuming food and beverages expected to cause heartburn, acid indigestion, or sour stomach. Pepcid AC and Tagamet HB also are labeled for relief of the symptoms. A fourth acid reducer, Zantac 75 (ranitidine hydrochloride), is labeled only for relief. The drugs are for people age 12 or older.

Users should take no more than four tablets of Tagamet HB or two tablets of the other acid reducers in 24 hours, and should limit use at the maximum dose without consulting a doctor to two weeks. They should consult a doctor if they have swallowing difficulty or persistent abdominal pain, as these symptoms may indicate a more serious condition.

In addition, with Tagamet HB, people should consult their doctors before use if they also take any of these prescription drugs: theophylline (oral asthma medicine), warfarin (blood-thinning medicine), or phenytoin (seizure medicine). If people have questions about whether their medicines contain these drugs or about other drug interactions, they should call the manufacturer, SmithKline Beecham Consumer Affairs, at (1-800) 482-4394.

Most products approved to relieve heartburn, indigestion, or upset stomach from too much food or drink are antacids, which neutralize gastric acidity.

Antacids may contain various active ingredients. The four general categories, with common brands and potential side effects, are:

- Sodium salts (Alka-Seltzer, Bromo Seltzer, and others)—People on salt-restricted diets, especially if being treated for high blood pressure, should only take sodium antacids under a doctor's orders. FDA requires labels of all OTC antacids to give the sodium content. Because a risk of stomach rupture has been associated with sodium bicarbonate intended to be dissolved in water, FDA has proposed a "Stomach Warning" in product labeling: "To avoid serious injury, do not take until [insert product dosage form, e.g., "tablet," "powder"] is completely dissolved. It is very important not to take this product when overly full from food or drink. Consult a doctor if severe stomach pain occurs after taking this product."

- Calcium salts (Alka-2, Rolaids [Calcium Rich], Titralac, Tums, and others)—Extended heavy use of calcium antacids (20 grams or more daily for a prolonged period) may cause excess calcium in the blood, which can lead to kidney stones and reduced kidney function. People who already have impaired kidneys may develop milk-alkali syndrome (causing symptoms such as nausea, vomiting, mental confusion, and loss of appetite) with as little as 4 grams a day.

- Aluminum salts (ALternaGEL, Amphogel, Rolaids, and others)—Aluminum salts can constipate, so they're usually combined with magnesium salts to counter this effect. Overuse can weaken bones, especially in people with impaired kidney function, leading to conditions such as osteomalacia (softening of the bones, which causes symptoms such as tenderness, muscular weakness, and weight loss).

- Magnesium salts (Camalox, Gelusil, Maalox, Mylanta, and others)—These salts have a laxative effect, so they're usually combined with aluminum salts; Camalox also has calcium salts. Very prolonged use may cause kidney stones. Too much magnesium in the blood can cause heart, central nervous system, and kidney problems.

As this list shows, some antacid products contain a combination of antacid ingredients. Some also contain simethicone, which breaks up gas bubbles, making them easier to eliminate from the body.

"Antacids are fast-acting drugs," says Hugo Gallo-Torres, M.D., a medical officer in FDA's division of gastrointestinal and coagulation drug products. "They should bring relief within 15 to 20 minutes of each episode. If, after several episodes, there is no relief, then something else may be going on, something that requires a physician's evaluation."

Antacids may interact with many drugs. Gallo-Torres advises consulting a doctor before using antacids if you have a condition that requires adjusting sodium in your diet, or if you are taking a prescription medicine.

Ways to Avoid Heartburn

The best way to deal with heartburn or indigestion is to avoid them in the first place. Simple preventive steps are:

- **Avoid big meals.** Your stomach must work long and hard to process them, which means it must produce a lot of acid. It helps to eat more frequent, smaller meals.

- **After you eat, don't lie down right away.** If you do, you're more likely to have heartburn, because gravity is now preventing food from going speedily to the intestines.

- **Eat your last full meal at least three hours before bedtime.** When you go to sleep, everything slows down, including your digestive system, so food you've eaten right before bedtime will stay in your stomach longer. It won't feel good.

- **Sleep with your head and shoulders propped up** 6 to 8 inches, so that your body is at a slight angle. This gets gravity working for you and not against you. Digestive juices in your stomach are then more likely to head south, for your intestines, instead of back up into your esophagus to cause a burning sensation.

- **Avoid tight-fitting garments.** They can literally compress your stomach, making it more likely that the stomach's acid contents will back up into your esophagus.

- **Avoid foods that contain a lot of acid,** such as citrus fruits and tomatoes, and any other food that gives you problems.

- **Cut down on caffeine.** It makes your stomach produce more acid. Caffeine-heavy items include coffee, tea, chocolate, and some sodas.

- **Cut down on alcohol and smoking.** Both irritate the lining of your stomach and tend to lower esophageal sphincter pressure. When this happens, it's easier for the stomach's acid contents to shoot back up your esophagus.

Overindulgence

Bismuth subsalicylate is recommended for overeating and drinking excessively. Bismuth also has some antibacterial effect. The product, sold as Pepto-Bismol and generic brands, may cause a temporary, harmless darkening of the tongue or stool.

FDA has proposed that products containing bismuth subsalicylate have labeling warning not to give the drug to children and teenagers who have or are recovering from chickenpox, flu symptoms (nausea, vomiting or fever), or flu. The warning is needed because, like aspirin, bismuth subsalicylate is a salicylate and may be associated with an increased risk of Reye syndrome, a rare but serious illness that can occur in children and teenagers with those illnesses.

Other proposed warnings advise users not to take the drug if they're allergic to any salicylate, and to consult a doctor first if they have diabetes, gout or arthritis, or if they take blood-thinning medicine.

Users are also advised to stop taking the drug if they have ringing in the ears. Rachanow explains: "This may happen when too much drug is taken or when another salicylate, such as aspirin, is taken at the same time."

Viral Infection

Nausea, vomiting and diarrhea may also be due to mild viral gastrointestinal infection. Children are especially susceptible. A doctor should be consulted if vomiting or diarrhea recur or persist, because dehydration or a chemical imbalance may result and require treatment. It is very important that patients recovering from viral gastrointestinal infection drink plenty of fluids.

General Advice

With stomach upsets in general, it's a good idea to call the doctor if symptoms last more than a few days. A doctor should be called if symptoms become severe-for instance:

- continuous vomiting or diarrhea
- extreme discomfort or pain in the gastrointestinal tract
- black stool (unless the drug you took, such as Pepto Bismol, contains bismuth subsalicylate)
- visible blood in the stool
- vomiting of blood or material that looks like coffee grounds, but which is actually digested blood.

Prolonged self-treatment may mask a more serious condition, such as an ulcer or cancer.

Women who are pregnant or breast-feeding should consult their doctors before taking any drugs.

Fortunately, most upset stomachs get better by themselves or require minimal treatment. As with any medicine, it's important to read an OTC drug's entire label and follow directions carefully. And, as with any illness, it's important to know when to call the doctor.

—by Dixie Farley

Dixie Farley is a staff writer for FDA Consumer.

Table 8.1. OTC Drugs for Upset Stomachs (continued on next page).

Motion Sickness (Antihistamines)

Drug: cyclizine
Common Brands: Marezine
Possible Side Effects: drowsiness; dry mouth; rarely, blurred vision

Drug: dimenhydrinate
Common Brands: Dramamine
Possible Side Effects: drowsiness; dry mouth; rarely, blurred vision

Drug: diphenhydramine
Common Brands: Benadryl
Possible Side Effects: drowsiness; dry mouth; rarely, blurred vision

Drug: meclizine
Common Brands: Bonine
Possible Side Effects: drowsiness; dry mouth; rarely, blurred vision

Heartburn, Indigestion, Sour Stomach (Antacids)

Drug: sodium salts
Common Brands: Alka-Seltzer, Bromo Seltzer
Possible Side Effects: interference with salt-restricted diet; with sodium bicarbonate to be dissolved in water, risk of stomach rupture if product is not fully dissolved

Drug: calcium salts
Common Brands: Alka-2, Calcium Rich, Rolaids, Titralac, Tums
Possible Side Effects: with extended heavy use, kidney stones, reduced kidney function

Drug: aluminum salts
Common Brands: ALternaGEL, Amphogel, Rolaids
Possible Side Effects: constipation; with overuse, weakened bones

Table 8.1. OTC Drugs for Upset Stomachs (continued from previous page).

> Drug: magnesium salts
>
> Common Brands: Camalox, Gelusil, Maalox, Mylanta
>
> Possible Side Effects: laxative effect; with prolonged use, kidney stones; with excessive blood magnesium, problems of the heart, central nervous system, and kidneys

Heartburn, Indigestion, Sour Stomach (Acid Reducers)

> Drug: famotidine
>
> Common Brands: Pepcid AC Acid Controller
>
> Possible Side Effects (seen at higher prescription dosages): headache, dizziness, constipation, diarrhea
>
> Drug: nizatidine
>
> Common Brands: Axid AR
>
> Possible Side Effects (seen at higher prescription dosages) headache, dizziness
>
> Drug: ranitidine hydrochloride
>
> Common Brands: Zantac 75
>
> Possible Side Effects (seen at higher prescription dosages): headache, constipation, diarrhea; elevated liver enzymes when given intravenously
>
> Drug: cimetidine
>
> Common Brands: Tagamet HB
>
> Possible Side Effects (seen at higher prescription dosages): headache, diarrhea, dizziness, sleepiness; Rx and OTC–drug interactions with theophylline, warfarin or phenytoin

Overindulgence

> Drug: bismuth subsalicylate
>
> Common Brands: Pepto-Bismol
>
> Possible Side Effects: temporary, harmless darkening of the tongue or stool; risk of Reye syndrome in children or teenagers who have or are recovering from flu or chickenpox; with overuse, ringing in the ears

Chapter 9

Steroid Use in Gastrointestinal Diseases

Corticosteroids are potent anti-inflammatory agents used in a wide range of diseases. In gastrointestinal disorders, steroids are primarily prescribed for the treatment of inflammatory bowel disease (e.g. ulcerative colitis or Crohn's disease), but are also used in such processes as autoimmune hepatitis, eosinophilic gastroenteritis, and other inflammatory conditions that involve the gastrointestinal tract. Steroids are quite effective at decreasing inflammation, but their use is limited by numerous side effects. Although this chapter will focus on inflammatory bowel disease (IBD), the principles are applicable to any intestinal disease treated with steroids.

When to Use Steroids

Often IBD responds well to agents that work on inflammation, e.g. sulfasalazine and mesalamine (Asacol, Pentasa), or agents that modulate the immune system, e.g. antibiotics (Cipro and Flagyl), 6-mercaptopurine (6MP) or Imuran. Steroids are required for patients who are not responding to these medicines or are having a particularly severe flare. A physician will make the decision to treat a patient with steroids based on symptoms, such as profuse diarrhea, bleeding, abdominal pain, or on endoscopic or radiologic testing that demonstrates severe intestinal inflammation.

"Steroid Use in GI Diseases," by Miguel Regueiro, MD, in *Intestinal Fortitude*, Vol. 9, Issue 2, 1998, © 1998 Intestinal Disease Foundation, 1322 Forbes Ave., Suite 200, Pittsburgh, PA 15219, (412) 261-5888; reprinted with permission.

How Steroids Are Prescribed

The administration of steroids can be either in the form of a pill that is ingested (e.g. prednisone) or an intravenous infusion (e.g. methylprednisolone). The choice of which route to administer the steroid depends entirely on the severity of disease. Patients who are admitted to the hospital for a severe IBD flare are usually started on intravenous steroids and then changed over to the oral form when they have improved. Steroids are discontinued when the patient is on a stable regimen of medicine, e.g. 6MP, mesalamine, or antibiotics, and has symptomatic improvement.

Steroids must be withdrawn slowly and should never be stopped suddenly. Steroids suppress the normal ability of the adrenal glands to produce the body's own steroid hormones. If steroids are discontinued abruptly adrenal crisis or insufficiency could result. The most common symptoms of adrenal insufficiency are weight loss, weakness, anorexia, low blood pressure, and fatigue. The usual course for stopping steroids varies from doctor to doctor, but always involves a slow taper over a period of time. An example of a steroid taper would be to decrease the dose by 10 mg. every 4-7 days until off completely; a patient that is on a dose of 40 mg. of prednisone a day would decrease to 30 mg. for one week, then 20 mg. for one week, then 10 mg. for one week, and then stop.

How Steroids Work

Steroids are potent anti-inflammatory agents that work through two mechanisms. They prevent the formation of inflammatory chemicals (arachidonic acid, prostaglandins, and leukotrienes) by inhibiting a specific enzyme (phospholipase A2). They also seem to have activity against certain parts of the immune system involved in inflammation (specifically, they inhibit IL-2 from activating helper T cells).

Steroids work quickly and patients having a severe flare of their IBD will often feel an improvement within days. Likewise, patients who have initially improved on steroids may notice a recurrence in symptoms when their dosage is tapered. To avoid a recurrent flare, a prolonged tapering period or the addition of an immunomodulator agent, such as 6MP, may be necessary.

Side Effects

As effective as steroids are at controlling a flare of IBD, their long-term usage is fraught with side effects. If limited to a short duration of treatment, steroids rarely cause serious adverse effects, even at high doses. The most common side effects from short-term therapy include fluid retention, hypertension, insomnia, mood alterations, electrolyte abnormalities (high glucose or low potassium levels), and stomach upset. Long-term use is associated with hirsutism (increased growth of hair), acne, obesity, striae ("stretch marks"), and potentially devastating effects, including impaired growth in children, osteoporosis (bone loss), aseptic necrosis, cataracts, diabetes, and muscle breakdown resulting in weakness. Almost all patients treated with steroids for a long period of time will develop some degree of adrenal suppression.

Steroids in Pregnancy

Patients with IBD "in remission" will often not have a flare of their disease during pregnancy. Nonetheless, IBD flares do occur during pregnancy and can lead to complications unless treated. The treatment of IBD during pregnancy is usually no different than in a non-pregnant patient. Despite the risks of long-term steroid use, the short-term use of steroids in pregnancy and during nursing is safe. Since the consequences of uncontrolled inflammation can be harmful to the fetus, steroids may be used at an earlier point, than would otherwise, in the treatment course. Regardless of the treatment, the management of IBD in pregnancy should be closely coordinated between the obstetrician and gastroenterologist.

Newer and Safer Steroids?

Within the past ten years rapidly metabolized steroids have been researched for a variety of inflammatory diseases. Rapidly metabolized steroids were developed because of their anti-inflammatory potential and theoretical lack of side effects. Rapidly metabolized steroids, including beclomethasone, tixocortol, fluticasone, and budesonide, are now under investigation for the treatment of IBD. Budesonide has received the most attention in recent studies and may be useful in the treatment of Crohn's disease. Unfortunately these agents are not yet available in this country and recent studies suggest that they may not be as safe or efficacious as once thought. Nonetheless, these agents still hold enormous potential for the treatment of IBD, and future trials in this country are anticipated.

Part Two

Digestive Diseases and Functional Disorders

Chapter 10

Appendicitis

About Appendicitis

Appendicitis is inflammation of the appendix, a small portion of the large intestine that hangs down from the lower right side. Although the appendix does not seem to serve any purpose, it can still become diseased. If untreated, an inflamed appendix can burst, causing infection and even death. About 1 in 500 people has appendicitis each year.

Appendicitis may occur after a viral infection in the digestive tract or when the tube connecting the large intestine and appendix is blocked by trapped stool. The inflammation can cause infection, a blood clot, or rupture of the appendix. Because of the risk of rupture, appendicitis is considered an emergency. Anyone with symptoms needs to see a doctor immediately. Symptoms include:

- Pain in the right side of the abdomen. The pain usually begins near the navel and moves down and to the right. The pain becomes worse when moving, taking deep breaths, coughing, sneezing, and being touched in the area.

- Nausea.

- Vomiting.

This chapter contains text from "Appendicitis," National Digestive Diseases Information Clearinghouse (NDIC), April 1998; and "About Appendectomy," American College of Surgeons, 55 East Erie Street, Chicago, IL, March 1994; reprinted with permission.

- Constipation.
- Diarrhea.
- Inability to pass gas.
- Low fever that begins after other symptoms.
- Abdominal swelling.

Not everyone has all symptoms. It is important that people with symptoms of appendicitis not take laxatives or enemas to relieve constipation because these medicines could cause the appendix to burst. People also should not take pain medicine because it can mask symptoms that the doctor needs to know about.

The doctor bases an appendicitis diagnosis on symptoms, a physical exam, blood tests to check for signs of infection such as a high white blood cell count, and urine tests to rule out a urinary tract infection. Some doctors use ultrasound to see whether the appendix looks inflamed. Treatment is surgery to remove the appendix, called appendectomy. Doctors are beginning to use laparoscopic surgery for appendectomy. This technique involves making several tiny cuts in the abdomen and inserting a miniature camera and surgical instruments. The surgeon then removes the appendix with the instruments, so there is no need to make a large incision in the abdomen. People can live a normal life without their appendix—no changes in diet, exercise, or other lifestyle factors are necessary.

About Appendectomy

Appendectomy (ap-pen-DECK-toe-me) is the surgical removal of the appendix. This section will explain to you:

- Why you may need to have an appendectomy
- The ways in which an appendix is removed
- What to expect before and after the operation

Remember, no two people undergoing an appendectomy are alike. The reasons for and the outcome of any surgical procedure depend on your age, the severity of your problem, and your general health. This chapter is not intended to take the place of your surgeon's professional opinion. Rather, it is intended to help you begin to understand the basics of this surgical procedure. Read this information carefully. If you have questions after reading this material, discuss them openly and honestly with your surgeon.

What Is the Appendix?

The appendix is a three- to six-inch long tubelike structure that projects from the junction of the small and large intestines. No one knows what, if any, function the appendix has. However, once the appendix becomes infected or inflamed, it must be removed. The appendix may vary in its orientation to the small intestine and the cecum (the expandable pouch in which the large intestine begins and into which the ileum opens from one side). Such variation can account for confusing and atypical symptoms that can make diagnosis difficult.

What Is Appendicitis?

Obstruction of the appendix by fecal matter or some other cause can lead to an inflammation of the appendix called appendicitis. Appendicitis usually develops rapidly with little warning over a period of six to 12 hours. The usual symptom is abdominal pain, which begins as vague discomfort around the navel. Over the next several hours, the pain becomes much more severe and is localized to the lower right side of the abdomen. The abdomen may become rigid and very sensitive to pressure. Pain is typically accompanied by nausea, vomiting and a slight fever.

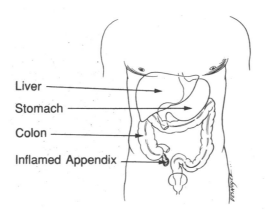

Figure 10.1. *Inflammation of the appendix is called appendicitis.*

Who Gets Appendicitis?

Approximately two-thirds of all people who experience appendicitis are women, and about two-thirds of all people who get appendicitis are between the ages of 15 and 44. However, this condition can affect any person, at any age.

Diagnosing Appendicitis

An appendectomy is almost always performed as emergency surgery. Therefore, a diagnosis of appendicitis is usually made swiftly and is based primarily on an analysis of your symptoms and a physical examination. If there is a question regarding the nature of your symptoms—or if the symptoms do not seem urgent, blood tests and an abdominal x-ray may be done. Preparations include the usual admission tests, including: complete blood count, blood clotting tests, urinalysis, and chest x-ray.

Preparing for Surgery

Because you are arriving at the hospital as an emergency admission, you will be asked how long it has been since you last consumed food. The reason for this question is that a general anesthetic, which is usually given to the patient before an appendectomy is performed, can only be given on an empty stomach.

You will receive a preoperative sedative by injection to make you sleepy. Also, an intravenous (IV) needle will be inserted into the back of your hand or forearm for connection to an IV line in the operating room through which the general anesthetic will be administered.

The entire procedure usually takes about one hour.

The Surgical Procedure

Today, a surgeon can perform an appendectomy in one of two ways: through what is called an open operation or through the laparoscopic technique.

The Open Technique. In this operation, the surgeon makes a short incision through the skin and underlying fat. The muscles of the wall are then separated, revealing the peritoneum, which is the lining of the abdominal cavity. The peritoneum is cut to reveal the cecum, the section of the large intestine to which the appendix is attached. After the small intestine has been moved aside, the appendix is carefully freed from the surrounding structures. Blood vessels around the site are tied off.

At this point, the appendix is tied off and severed. The appendix is then sent to the pathology laboratory for examination. The stump of the appendix is positioned into the cecum. Finally, the peritoneum, the muscle wall, and the skin incision are closed. Closure of the skin is done either with sutures or tiny staples.

The Laparoscopic Technique. A laparoscope is used to view the inside of the abdominal cavity while the surgeon removes the appendix. A laparoscope is a long metal tube with a lens on which a TV camera is attached. The surgeon can then perform the appendectomy directly from the TV monitor. Surgical instruments called cannulas are inserted into other small openings and used to remove the appendix. Laparoscopic appendectomy is a safe alternative to the open technique. Presently, there seems to be no difference between the two techniques in terms of hospital costs, length of the patient's hospital stay, or infection rate. It may, however, let patients resume normal activity more quickly than the open technique permits. This method is not for every patient, and it is up to you and your surgeon to decide whether it is right for you.

Regardless of the type of procedure you undergo, minimal postoperative discomfort is likely to occur after an appendectomy. You will be given oral medication for any discomfort you may experience.

Recovery from the Operation

You will remain in the recovery room for about one hour after your appendectomy. If you had an open appendectomy, you will be up and walking within six hours. Expect to be discharged from the hospital—barring complications—in one to two days.

If you have a laparoscopy, you will most likely be discharged on the day of your operation.

Your doctor may instruct you to refrain from jogging and lifting heavy objects for one to several weeks, depending on the type and complexity of your operation.

What about Complications?

Complications are rare following an appendectomy. However, if the appendix ruptures before surgery, peritonitis, a potentially life-threatening infection of the abdominal cavity, may occur. Treatment then will include intravenous administration of antibiotics to control the infection. Some patients who are suspected to have appendicitis, even though they have no symptoms, may undergo an appendectomy to ensure that rupture of the appendix and other complications are avoided.

Will I Have a Scar?

You will have a short scar at the location of the incision. Typically, the scar is placed in a natural fold just above the groin and is very inconspicuous.

Reviewed by

J. Barry McKernan, MD, Ph.D., F.A.C.S., Clinical Professor of Surgery, Medical College of Georgia, Augusta and Emory University, Atlanta.

George F. Sheldon, MD, F.A.C.S., Professor and Chairman, Department of Surgery, University of North Carolina, Chapel Hill.

Surgery by Surgeons

A fully trained surgeon is a physician who, after medical school, has gone through years of training in an accredited residency program to learn the specialized skills of a surgeon. One good sign of a surgeon's competence is certification by a national surgical board approved by the American Board of Medical Specialties. All board-certified surgeons have satisfactorily completed an approved residency training program and have passed a rigorous specialty examination.

The letters F.A.C.S. (Fellow of the American College of Surgeons) after a surgeon's name are a further indication of a physician's qualifications. Surgeons who become Fellows of the College have passed a comprehensive evaluation of their surgical training and skills; they also have demonstrated their commitment to high standards of ethical conduct. This evaluation is conducted according to national standards that were established to ensure that patients receive the best possible surgical care.

Prepared as a public service by the American College of Surgeons.

American College of Surgeons
55 East Eric Street
Chicago, IL 60611

Chapter 11

Bleeding in the Digestive Tract

Introduction

Bleeding in the digestive tract is a symptom of digestive problems rather than a disease itself. Bleeding can occur as the result of a number of different conditions, many of which are not life threatening. Most causes of bleeding are related to conditions that can be cured or controlled, such as hemorrhoids. The cause of bleeding may not be serious, but locating the source of bleeding is important.

The digestive or gastrointestinal (GI) tract includes the esophagus, stomach, small intestine, large intestine or colon, rectum, and anus. Bleeding can come from one or more of these areas, that is, from a small area such as an ulcer on the lining of the stomach or from a large surface such as an inflammation of the colon. Bleeding can sometimes occur without the person noticing it. This type of bleeding is called occult or hidden. Fortunately, simple tests can detect occult blood in the stool.

Questions and Answers about Bleeding in the Digestive Tract

What Causes Bleeding in the Digestive Tract?

Stomach acid can cause inflammation that may lead to bleeding at the lower end of the esophagus. This condition is called esophagitis

National Institute of Diabetes and Digestive and Kidney Diseases (NIDDK), NIH Publication No. 95-1133, updated November 1998.

or inflammation of the esophagus. Sometimes a muscle between the esophagus and stomach fails to close properly and allows the return of food and stomach juices into the esophagus, which can lead to esophagitis. In addition, enlarged veins (varices) at the lower end of the esophagus may rupture and bleed massively. Cirrhosis of the liver is the most common cause of esophageal varices. Esophageal bleeding can be caused by Mallory-Weiss syndrome, a tear in the lining of the esophagus. Mallory-Weiss syndrome usually results from prolonged vomiting but may also be caused by increased pressure in the abdomen from coughing, hiatal hernia, or childbirth.

The stomach is a frequent site of bleeding. Alcohol, aspirin, aspirin-containing medicines, and various other medicines (particularly those used for arthritis) can cause stomach ulcers or inflammation (gastritis). The stomach is often the site of ulcer disease. Acute or chronic ulcers may enlarge and erode through a blood vessel, causing bleeding. Also, patients suffering from burns, shock, head injuries, or cancer, or those who have undergone extensive surgery may develop stress ulcers. Bleeding can occur from benign tumors or cancer of the stomach, although these disorders usually do not cause massive bleeding.

The most common source of bleeding from the upper digestive tract is ulcers in the duodenum (the upper small intestine). Researchers now believe that these ulcers are caused by excess stomach acid and infection with *Helicobacter pylori* bacteria.

In the lower digestive tract, the large intestine and rectum are frequent sites of bleeding. Hemorrhoids are probably the most common cause of visible blood in the digestive tract, especially blood that appears bright red. Hemorrhoids are enlarged veins in the anal area that can rupture and produce bright red blood, which can show up in the toilet or on toilet paper. If red blood is seen, however, it is essential to exclude other causes of bleeding since the anal area may also be the site of cuts (fissures), inflammation, or tumors.

Benign growths or polyps of the colon are very common and are thought to be forerunners of cancer. These growths can cause either bright red blood or occult bleeding. Colorectal cancer is the second most frequent of all cancers in the United States and usually causes bleeding at some time.

Inflammation from various causes can produce extensive bleeding from the colon. Different intestinal infections can cause inflammation and bloody diarrhea. Ulcerative colitis can produce inflammation and extensive surface bleeding from tiny ulcerations. Crohn's disease of the large intestine can also produce spotty bleeding.

Diverticular disease caused by diverticula—outpouchings of the colon wall—can result in massive bleeding. Finally, as one gets older, abnormalities may develop in the blood vessels of the large intestine, which may result in recurrent bleeding.

What Are the Common Causes of Bleeding in the Digestive Tract?

Esophagus

- Inflammation (esophagitis)
- Enlarged veins (varices)
- Mallory-Weiss syndrome

Stomach

- Ulcers
- Inflammation (gastritis)

Small Intestine

- Duodenal ulcer

Large Intestine and Rectum

- IIemorrhoids
- Inflammation (ulcerative colitis)
- Colorectal polyps
- Colorectal cancer
- Diverticular disease

How Is Bleeding in the Digestive Tract Recognized?

The signs of bleeding in the digestive tract depend upon the site and severity of bleeding. If blood is coming from the rectum or the lower colon, bright red blood will coat or mix with the stool. The stool may be mixed with darker blood if the bleeding is higher up in the colon or at the far end of the small intestine. When there is bleeding in the esophagus, stomach, or duodenum, the stool is usually black or tarry. Vomited material may be bright red or have a coffee-grounds appearance when one is bleeding from those sites. If bleeding is occult, the patient might not notice any changes in stool color.

If sudden massive bleeding occurs, a person may feel weak, dizzy, faint, short of breath, or have crampy abdominal pain or diarrhea.

Shock may occur, with a rapid pulse, drop in blood pressure, and difficulty in producing urine. The patient may become very pale. If bleeding is slow and occurs over a long period of time, a gradual onset of fatigue, lethargy, shortness of breath, and pallor from the anemia will result. Anemia is a condition in which the blood's iron-rich substance, hemoglobin, is diminished.

How Is Bleeding in the Digestive Tract Diagnosed?

The site of the bleeding must be located. A complete history and physical examination are essential. Symptoms such as changes in bowel habits, stool color (to black or red) and consistency, and the presence of pain or tenderness may tell the doctor which area of the GI tract is affected. Because the intake of iron or foods such as beets can give the stool the same appearance as bleeding from the digestive tract, a doctor must test the stool for blood before offering a diagnosis. A blood count will indicate whether the patient is anemic and also will give an idea of the extent of the bleeding and how chronic it may be.

Endoscopy. Endoscopy is a common diagnostic technique that allows direct viewing of the bleeding site. Because the endoscope can detect lesions and confirm the presence or absence of bleeding, doctors often choose this method to diagnose patients with acute bleeding. In many cases, the doctor can use the endoscope to treat the cause of bleeding as well.

The endoscope is a flexible instrument that can be inserted through the mouth or rectum. The instrument allows the doctor to see into the esophagus, stomach, duodenum (esophago-duodenoscopy), colon (colonoscopy), and rectum (sigmoidoscopy); to collect small samples of tissue (biopsies); to take photographs; and to stop the bleeding.

Small bowel endoscopy, or enteroscopy, is a new procedure using a long endoscope. This endoscope may be introduced during surgery to localize a source of bleeding in the small intestine.

Other Procedures. Several other methods are available to locate the source of bleeding. Barium x-rays, in general, are less accurate than endoscopy in locating bleeding sites. Some drawbacks of barium x-rays are that they may interfere with other diagnostic techniques if used for detecting acute bleeding; they expose the patient to x-rays; and they do not offer the capabilities of biopsy or treatment.

Angiography is a technique that uses dye to highlight blood vessels. This procedure is most useful in situations when the patient is acutely bleeding such that dye leaks out of the blood vessel and identifies the site of bleeding. In selected situations, angiography allows injection of medicine into arteries that may stop the bleeding.

Radionuclide scanning is a noninvasive screening technique used for locating sites of acute bleeding, especially in the lower GI tract. This technique involves injection of small amounts of radioactive material. Then, a special camera produces pictures of organs, allowing the doctor to detect a bleeding site.

In addition, barium x-rays, angiography, and radionuclide scans can be used to locate sources of chronic occult bleeding. These techniques are especially useful when the small intestine is suspected as the site of bleeding since the small intestine may not be seen easily with endoscopy.

How Is Bleeding in the Digestive Tract Treated?

The use of endoscopy has grown and now allows doctors not only to see bleeding sites but to directly apply therapy as well. A variety of endoscopic therapies are useful to the patient for treating GI tract bleeding.

Active bleeding from the upper GI tract can often be controlled by injecting chemicals directly into a bleeding site with a needle introduced through the endoscope. A physician can also cauterize, or heat treat, a bleeding site and surrounding tissue with a heater probe or electrocoagulation device passed through the endoscope. Laser therapy, although effective, is no longer used regularly by many physicians because it is expensive and cumbersome.

Once bleeding is controlled, medicines are often prescribed to prevent recurrence of bleeding. Medical treatment of ulcers to ensure healing and maintenance therapy to prevent ulcer recurrence can also lessen the chance of recurrent bleeding. Studies are now under way to see if elimination of *Helicobacter pylori* affects the recurrence of ulcer bleeding.

Removal of polyps with an endoscope can control bleeding from colon polyps. Removal of hemorrhoids by banding or various heat or electrical devices is effective in patients who suffer hemorrhoidal bleeding on a recurrent basis. Endoscopic injection or cautery can be used to treat bleeding sites throughout the lower intestinal tract.

Endoscopic techniques do not always control bleeding. Sometimes angiography may be used. However, surgery is often needed to control active, severe, or recurrent bleeding when endoscopy is not successful.

How Do You Recognize Blood in the Stool and Vomit?

- Bright red blood coating the stool
- Dark blood mixed with the stool
- Black or tarry stool
- Bright red blood in vomit
- Coffee-grounds appearance of vomit

What Are the Symptoms of Acute Bleeding?

- Weakness
- Shortness of breath
- Dizziness
- Crampy abdominal pain
- Faintness
- Diarrhea

What Are the Symptoms of Chronic Bleeding?

- Fatigue
- Shortness of breath
- Lethargy
- Pallor

Chapter 12

Celiac Disease

What Is Celiac Disease?

Celiac disease is a digestive disease that damages the small intestine and interferes with absorption of nutrients from food. People who have celiac disease cannot tolerate a protein called gluten, which is found in wheat, rye, barley, and possibly oats. When people with celiac disease eat foods containing gluten, their immune system responds by damaging the small intestine. Specifically, tiny fingerlike protrusions, called villi, on the lining of the small intestine are lost. Nutrients from food are absorbed into the bloodstream through these villi. Without villi, a person becomes malnourished—regardless of the quantity of food eaten.

Because the body's own immune system causes the damage, celiac disease is considered an autoimmune disorder. However, it is also classified as a disease of malabsorption because nutrients are not absorbed. Celiac disease is also known as celiac sprue, nontropical sprue, and gluten-sensitive enteropathy.

Celiac disease is a genetic disease, meaning that it runs in families. Sometimes the disease is triggered—or becomes active for the first time—after surgery, pregnancy, childbirth, viral infection, or severe emotional stress.

National Institute of Diabetes and Digestive and Kidney Diseases (NIDDK), NIH Publication No. 98-4225, April 1998.

What Are the Symptoms?

Celiac disease affects people differently. Some people develop symptoms as children, others as adults. One factor thought to play a role in when and how celiac appears is whether and how long a person was breastfed—the longer one was breastfed, the later symptoms of celiac disease appear, and the more atypical the symptoms. Other factors include the age at which one began eating foods containing gluten and how much gluten is eaten.

Symptoms may or may not occur in the digestive system. For example, one person might have diarrhea and abdominal pain, while another person has irritability or depression. In fact, irritability is one of the most common symptoms in children.

Symptoms of celiac disease may include one or more of the following:

- Recurring abdominal bloating and pain.
- Chronic diarrhea.
- Weight loss.
- Pale, foul-smelling stool.
- Unexplained anemia (low count of red blood cells).
- Gas.
- Bone pain.
- Behavior changes.
- Muscle cramps.
- Fatigue.
- Delayed growth.
- Failure to thrive in infants.
- Pain in the joints.
- Seizures.
- Tingling numbness in the legs (from nerve damage)
- Pale sores inside the mouth, called aphthus ulcers.
- Painful skin rash, called dermatitis herpetiformis.
- Tooth discoloration or loss of enamel.
- Missed menstrual periods (often because of excessive weight loss).

Anemia, delayed growth, and weight loss are signs of malnutrition—not getting enough nutrients. Malnutrition is a serious problem for anyone, but particularly for children because they need adequate nutrition to develop properly.

Some people with celiac disease may not have symptoms. The undamaged part of their small intestine is able to absorb enough nutrients to prevent symptoms. However, people without symptoms are still at risk for complications of celiac disease. (Complications are described below.)

How Is Celiac Disease Diagnosed?

Diagnosing celiac disease can be difficult because some of its symptoms are similar to those of other diseases, including irritable bowel syndrome, Crohn's disease, ulcerative colitis, diverticulosis, intestinal infections, chronic fatigue syndrome, and depression.

Recently, researchers discovered that people with celiac disease have higher than normal levels of certain antibodies in their blood. Antibodies are produced by the immune system in response to substances that the body perceives to be threatening. To diagnose celiac disease, physicians test blood to measure levels of antibodies to gluten. These antibodies are antigliadin, anti-endomysium, and antireticulin.

If the tests and symptoms suggest celiac disease, the physician may remove a tiny piece of tissue from the small intestine to check for damage to the villi. This is done in a procedure called a biopsy: the physician eases a long, thin tube called an endoscope through the mouth and stomach into the small intestine, and then takes a sample of tissue using instruments passed through the endoscope. Biopsy of the small intestine is the best way to diagnose celiac disease.

Screening

Screening for celiac disease involves testing asymptomatic people for the antibodies to gluten. Americans are not routinely screened for celiac disease. However, because celiac disease is hereditary, family members—particularly first-degree relatives—of people who have been diagnosed may need to be tested for the disease. About 10 percent of an affected person's first-degree relatives (parents, siblings, or children) will also have the disease. The longer a person goes undiagnosed and untreated, the greater the chance of developing malnutrition and other complications.

What Is the Treatment?

The only treatment for celiac disease is to follow a gluten-free diet—that is, to avoid all foods that contain gluten. For most people, following this diet will stop symptoms, heal existing intestinal damage, and prevent further damage. Improvements begin within days of starting the diet, and the small intestine is usually completely healed—meaning the villi are intact and working—in 3 to 6 months. (It may take up to 2 years for older adults.)

The gluten-free diet is a lifetime requirement. Eating any gluten, no matter how small an amount, can damage the intestine. This is true for anyone with the disease, including people who do not have noticeable symptoms. Depending on a person's age at diagnosis, some problems, such as delayed growth and tooth discoloration, may not improve.

A small percentage of people with celiac disease do not improve on the gluten-free diet. These people often have severely damaged intestines that cannot heal even after they eliminate gluten from their diets. Because their intestines are not absorbing enough nutrients, they may need to receive intravenous nutrition supplements. Drug treatments are being evaluated for unresponsive celiac disease. These patients may need to be evaluated for complications of the disease.

If a person responds to the gluten-free diet, the physician will know for certain that the diagnosis of celiac disease is correct.

The Gluten-Free Diet

A gluten-free diet means avoiding all foods that contain wheat (including spelt, triticale, and kamut), rye, barley, and possibly oats—in other words, most grain, pasta, cereal, and many processed foods. Despite these restrictions, people with celiac disease can eat a well-balanced diet with a variety of foods, including bread and pasta. For example, instead of wheat flour, people can use potato, rice, soy, or bean flour. Or, they can buy gluten-free bread, pasta, and other products from special food companies.

Whether people with celiac disease should avoid oats is controversial because some people have been able to eat oats without having a reaction. Scientists are doing studies to find out whether people with celiac disease can tolerate oats. Until the studies are complete, people with celiac disease should follow their physician or dietitian's advice about eating oats.

Plain meat, fish, rice, fruits, and vegetables do not contain gluten, so people with celiac disease can eat as much of these foods as they like.

The gluten-free diet is complicated. It requires a completely new approach to eating that affects a person's entire life. People with celiac disease have to be extremely careful about what they buy for lunch at school or work, eat at cocktail parties, or grab from the refrigerator for a midnight snack. Eating out can be a challenge as the person with celiac disease learns to scrutinize the menu for foods with gluten and question the waiter or chef about possible hidden sources of gluten. However, with practice, screening for gluten becomes second nature and people learn to recognize which foods are safe and which are off limits.

A dietitian, a health care professional who specializes in food and nutrition, can help people learn about their new diet. Also, support groups are particularly helpful for newly diagnosed people and their families as they learn to adjust to a new way of life.

What Are the Complications of Celiac Disease?

Damage to the small intestine and the resulting problems with nutrient absorption put a person with celiac disease at risk for several diseases and health problems.

- Lymphoma and adenocarcinoma are types of cancer that can develop in the intestine.

- Osteoporosis is a condition in which the bones become weak, brittle, and prone to breaking. Poor calcium absorption is a contributing factor to osteoporosis.

- Miscarriage and congenital malformation of the baby, such as neural tube defects, are risks for untreated pregnant women with celiac disease because of malabsorption of nutrients.

- Short stature results when childhood celiac disease prevents nutrient absorption during the years when nutrition is critical to a child's normal growth and development. Children who are diagnosed and treated before their growth stops may have a catch-up period.

- Seizures, or convulsions, result from inadequate absorption of folic acid. Lack of folic acid causes calcium deposits, called calcifications, to form in the brain, which in turn cause seizures.

How Common Is Celiac Disease?

Celiac disease is the most common genetic disease in Europe. In Italy about 1 in 250 people and in Ireland about 1 in 300 people have celiac disease. It is rarely diagnosed in African, Chinese, and Japanese people.

An estimated 1 in 4,700 Americans have been diagnosed with celiac disease. Some researchers question how celiac disease could be so uncommon in the United States since it is hereditary and many Americans descend from European ethnic groups in whom the disease is common. A recent study in which random blood samples from the Red Cross were tested for celiac disease suggests that as many as 1 in every 250 Americans may have it. Celiac disease could be underdiagnosed in the United States for a number of reasons:

- Celiac symptoms can be attributed to other problems.
- Many doctors are not knowledgeable about the disease.
- Only a handful of U.S. laboratories are experienced and skilled in testing for celiac disease.

More research is needed to find out the true prevalence of celiac disease among Americans.

Diseases Linked to Celiac Disease

People with celiac disease tend to have other autoimmune diseases as well, including:

- Dermatitis herpetiformis.
- Thyroid disease.
- Systemic lupus erythematosus.
- Insulin-dependent diabetes.
- Liver disease.
- Collagen vascular disease.
- Rheumatoid arthritis.
- Sjogren's syndrome.

The connection between celiac and these diseases may be genetic.

Dermatitis Herpetiformis

Dermatitis herpetiformis (DH) is a severe itchy, blistering skin disease caused by gluten intolerance. DH is related to celiac disease since both are autoimmune disorders caused by gluten intolerance, but they are separate diseases. The rash usually occurs on the elbows, knees, and buttocks.

Although people with DH do not usually have digestive symptoms, they often have the same intestinal damage as people with celiac disease.

DH is diagnosed by a skin biopsy, which involves removing a tiny piece of skin near the rash and testing it for the IgA antibody. DH is treated with a gluten-free diet and medication to control the rash, such as dapsone or sulfapyridine. Drug treatment may last several years.

Additional Resources

American Celiac Society
58 Musano Court
West Orange, NJ 07052
(201) 325-8837

Celiac Disease Foundation
3251 Ventura Boulevard, #1
Studio City, CA 91604-1838
(818) 990-2354
Website: http://www.celiac.org/cdf
E-mail: cdf@primenet.com

Celiac Sprue Association/USA Inc.
P.O. Box 31700
Omaha, NE 68131-0700
(402) 558-0600
Website: http://www.csaceliacs.org/

Gluten Intolerance Group of North America
P.O. Box 23053
Seattle, WA 98102-0353
(206) 325-6980

National Center for Nutrition and Dietetics
American Dietetic Association
216 West Jackson Boulevard, Suite 800
Chicago, IL 60606-6995
(800) 366-1655

Gluten-Free Living *(a bimonthly newsletter)*
P.O. Box 105
Hastings-on-Hudson, NY 10706

Chapter 13

Colostomy

A New Beginning

Now that you have, or will have a colostomy, you are probably concerned about the changes in your life your surgery will cause. You may have some old-fashioned ideas about ostomy surgery or think there are only a few people in the world in your situation.

You should know that there are more than a million people in the United States and Canada with ostomies. They are working, playing and enjoying life just as they did before their surgery. Some are famous professional athletes, politicians and entertainers! Odds are, you have been in elevators with people with ostomies, worked with them, or played softball with them in your local league.

Think for a minute. Because a colostomy doesn't show, it can be kept a secret if you wish. Some of your best friends may have one, but you would know only if they told you.

Some Facts about Your Surgery

A colostomy is an opening in the abdominal wall through which digested food passes. A colostomy may be performed when a diseased or injured colon cannot be treated successfully with medicine.

When certain conditions are present in the lower bowel, it may be necessary to give that portion a rest by preventing feces from reaching it. To do this, a temporary colostomy is created by bringing a portion of the intestine through the abdominal wall to form a stoma on the abdomen. When you look at a stoma, you are actually looking at the lining of the intestine, which is like the lining of your cheek warm, moist and pink. In a temporary colostomy, when healing has taken place, the colostomy is eventually reversed (removed) and normal bowel movements are restored.

When the end portion of the colon or the rectum is diseased, construction of a permanent colostomy becomes necessary. A permanent colostomy usually involves the removal of part of the colon and in most cases, the rectum.

The end portion of the remaining colon is then brought through the abdominal wall to form a stoma.

Digested food, which passes through the stoma, is collected in a device called pouch or an appliance. The difference between today's ostomy pouches and those of the past is like the difference between night and day. Appliances today are not bulky and do not show under even the most stylish, form-fitting apparel for men and women. Whatever you wore before surgery, you can wear afterward with very few exceptions.

Pouches are odor-free and come in a variety of disposable or reusable varieties to fit your lifestyle. You are fitted for an appliance just as you are fitted for shoes or eyeglasses. Ostomy supplies are readily available at drug stores, ostomy supply houses, or through the mail.

Different types of colostomies are appropriate for different medical situations. One thing is true, however, no matter what the procedure, it is neither as difficult nor as unpleasant to live with a colostomy as you probably imagine.

Life with a Colostomy

You will not have to change to a new way of life, merely a new way of going to the bathroom. Adjusting to this change may seem frustrating at first, but be patient. It may take several months to complete your adjustment and reach the stage where your colostomy is just a minor inconvenience. At first, you may find yourself spending a great amount of time in the bathroom until you become proficient with the management of your ostomy. Once you have things down pat, your routine will speed up.

Work?

With the possible exception of jobs requiring very heavy lifting, your colostomy should not interfere with your work. People with colostomies are successful business people, taxi drivers, welders, sales people, carpenters, teachers, etc.

Sex and Social Life?

Physically, the creation of a colostomy usually does not affect sexual function. If there is a problem, it is almost always related to the removal of the rectum.

The colostomy itself should not interfere with pregnancy, and the risk during childbirth appears no greater than the risk for other women. An ostomy does not prevent one from dating, marriage, or having children. It will probably seem bigger and more important to you than to anyone else, including your boyfriend, girlfriend, lover, spouse, or children. Individuals with ostomies don't look different or smell bad, so your social life depends mainly on your attitude and personality.

Sports and Activities?

You can take a bath or shower with or without your pouch. Normal exposure to air or contact with soap and water will not harm your stoma. With a securely attached pouch, you can swim, camp out, climb mountains, play baseball or enjoy any other sport. (Consult your physician about heavy body-contact sports.)

You Are Not Alone

Your physician and hospital professionals are your first source of help for the many questions you have about your surgery. They can refer you to an enterostomal therapy (ET) nurse who is specially trained to help you learn to manage your stoma. They also can refer you to the United Ostomy Association (UOA) chapter in your area.

The UOA is a group of approximately 40,000 people with ostomies throughout the United States and Canada who have organized to help each other. The UOA publishes its own magazine, the *Ostomy Quarterly*, which provides updated ostomy information. It also sponsors educational conferences. Your local UOA chapter can provide an ostomy visitor who will be selected to suit your age, sex and type of ostomy.

It is very reassuring to talk with someone who has already been through the things you are reading about here.

The UOA has a library of publications offering more detailed information on ostomy, particularly *Colostomy: A Guide*. Publications cover topics such as colostomy management, employment, sex, children, and ostomy and many others. For information on the UOA, your local chapter, or a list of UOA publications, please call or write us at the address below. Good luck, and remember, you are not alone.

United Ostomy Association, Inc.
19772 MacArthur Blvd., Suite 200
Irvine, CA 92612-2405
(800) 826-0826
www.uoa.org
E-mail uoa@deltanet.com

Chapter 14

Constipation

Introduction

Constipation is passage of small amounts of hard, dry bowel movements, usually fewer than three times a week. People who are constipated may find it difficult and painful to have a bowel movement. Other symptoms of constipation include feeling bloated, uncomfortable, and sluggish.

Many people think they are constipated when, in fact, their bowel movements are regular. For example, some people believe they are constipated, or irregular, if they do not have a bowel movement every day. However, there is no right number of daily or weekly bowel movements. Normal may be three times a day or three times a week depending on the person. In addition, some people naturally have firmer stools than others.

At one time or another almost everyone gets constipated. Poor diet and lack of exercise are usually the causes. In most cases, constipation is temporary and not serious. Understanding causes, prevention, and treatment will help most people find relief.

Questions and Answers about Constipation

Who Gets Constipated?

According to the 1991 National Health Interview Survey, about 4½ million people in the United States say they are constipated most or

National Institute of Diabetes and Digestive and Kidney Diseases (NIDDK), NIH Pub. No. 95-2754, updated November 1998.

all of the time. Those reporting constipation most often are women, children, and adults age 65 and over. Pregnant women also complain of constipation, and it is a common problem following childbirth or surgery.

Constipation is the most common gastrointestinal complaint in the United States, resulting in about 2 million annual visits to the doctor. However, most people treat themselves without seeking medical help, as is evident from the $725 million Americans spend on laxatives each year.

What Causes Constipation?

To understand constipation, it helps to know how the colon (large intestine) works. As food moves through it, the colon absorbs water while forming waste products, or stool. Muscle contractions in the colon push the stool toward the rectum. By the time stool reaches the rectum, it is solid because most of the water has been absorbed. (See Figure 14.1.)

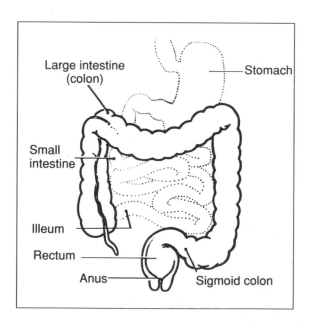

Figure 14.1. *Muscle contractions in the colon push the stool toward the rectum.*

The hard and dry stools of constipation occur when the colon absorbs too much water. This happens because the colon's muscle contractions are slow or sluggish, causing the stool to move through the colon too slowly. The most common causes of constipation are:

- Not enough fiber in the diet
- Not enough liquids
- Lack of exercise
- Medications
- Irritable bowel syndrome
- Changes in life or routine such as pregnancy, older age, and travel
- Abuse of laxatives
- Ignoring the urge to have a bowel movement
- Specific diseases such as multiple sclerosis and lupus
- Problems with the colon and rectum
- Problems with intestinal function (chronic idiopathic constipation)

Diet. The most common cause of constipation is a diet low in fiber found in vegetables, fruits, and whole grains and high in fats found in cheese, eggs, and meats. People who eat plenty of high-fiber foods are less likely to become constipated.

Fiber—soluble and insoluble—is the part of fruits, vegetables, and grains that the body cannot digest. Soluble fiber dissolves easily in water and takes on a soft, gel-like texture in the intestines. Insoluble fiber passes almost unchanged through the intestines. The bulk and soft texture of fiber help prevent hard, dry stools that are difficult to pass.

On average, Americans eat about 5 to 20 grams of fiber daily, short of the 20 to 35 grams recommended by the American Dietetic Association. Both children and adults eat too many refined and processed foods in which the natural fiber is removed.

A low-fiber diet also plays a key role in constipation among older adults. They often lack interest in eating and may choose fast foods low in fiber. In addition, loss of teeth may force older people to eat soft foods that are processed and low in fiber.

Not Enough Liquids. Liquids like water and juice add fluid to the colon and bulk to stools, making bowel movements softer and easier to pass. People who have problems with constipation should drink enough of these liquids every day, about eight 8-ounce glasses. Other liquids, like coffee and soft drinks, that contain caffeine seem to have a dehydrating effect.

Lack of Exercise. Lack of exercise can lead to constipation, although doctors do not know precisely why. For example, constipation often occurs after an accident or during an illness when one must stay in bed and cannot exercise.

Medications. Pain medications (especially narcotics), antacids that contain aluminum, antispasmodics, antidepressants, iron supplements, diuretics, and anticonvulsants for epilepsy can slow passage of bowel movements.

Irritable Bowel Syndrome (IBS). Some people with IBS, also known as spastic colon, have spasms in the colon that affect bowel movements. Constipation and diarrhea often alternate, and abdominal cramping, gassiness, and bloating are other common complaints. Although IBS can produce lifelong symptoms, it is not a life-threatening condition. It often worsens with stress, but there is no specific cause or anything unusual that the doctor can see in the colon.

Changes in Life or Routine. During pregnancy, women may be constipated because of hormonal changes or because the heavy uterus compresses the intestine. Aging may also affect bowel regularity because a slower metabolism results in less intestinal activity and muscle tone. In addition, people often become constipated when traveling because their normal diet and daily routines are disrupted.

Abuse of Laxatives. Myths about constipation have led to a serious abuse of laxatives. This is common among older adults who are preoccupied with having a daily bowel movement.

Laxatives usually are not necessary and can be habit-forming. The colon begins to rely on laxatives to bring on bowel movements. Over time, laxatives can damage nerve cells in the colon and interfere with the colon's natural ability to contract. For the same reason, regular use of enemas can also lead to a loss of normal bowel function.

Ignoring the Urge to Have a Bowel Movement. People who ignore the urge to have a bowel movement may eventually stop feeling the urge, which can lead to constipation. Some people delay having a bowel movement because they do not want to use toilets outside the home. Others ignore the urge because of emotional stress or because they are too busy. Children may postpone having a bowel movement because of stressful toilet training or because they do not want to interrupt their play.

Specific Diseases. Diseases that cause constipation include neurological disorders, metabolic and endocrine disorders, and systemic conditions that affect organ systems. These disorders can slow the movement of stool through the colon, rectum, or anus. The following diseases can cause constipation:

- Neurological disorders that may cause constipation include:

  - Multiple sclerosis
  - Parkinson's disease
  - Chronic idiopathic intestinal pseudo-obstruction
  - Stroke
  - Spinal cord injuries.

- Metabolic and endocrine conditions include:

  - Diabetes
  - Underactive or overactive thyroid gland
  - Uremia.

- Systemic disorders include:

  - Amyloidosis
  - Lupus
  - Scleroderma.

Problems with the Colon and Rectum. Intestinal obstruction, scar tissue (adhesions), diverticulosis, tumors, colorectal stricture, Hirschsprung's disease, or cancer can compress, squeeze, or narrow the intestine and rectum and cause constipation.

Problems with Intestinal Function (Chronic Idiopathic Constipation). Also known as functional constipation, chronic idiopathic (of unknown origin) constipation is rare. However, some people are chronically constipated and do not respond to standard treatment. This chronic constipation may be related to multiple problems with hormonal control or with nerves and muscles in the colon, rectum, or anus. Functional constipation occurs in both children and adults and is most common in women.

Colonic inertia and delayed transit are two types of functional constipation caused by decreased muscle activity in the colon. These syndromes may affect the entire colon or may be confined to the left or lower (sigmoid) colon.

Functional constipation that stems from abnormalities in the structure of the anus and rectum is known as anorectal dysfunction, or anismus. These abnormalities result in an inability to relax the rectal and anal muscles that allow stool to exit.

What Diagnostic Tests Are Used?

Most people do not need extensive testing and can be treated with changes in diet and exercise. For example, in young people with mild symptoms, a medical history and physical examination may be all the doctor needs to suggest successful treatment. The tests the doctor performs depends on the duration and severity of the constipation, the person's age, and whether there is blood in stools, recent changes in bowel movements, or weight loss.

Medical History. The doctor may ask a patient to describe his or her constipation, including duration of symptoms, frequency of bowel movements, consistency of stools, presence of blood in the stool, and toilet habits (how often and where one has bowel movements). Recording eating habits, medication, and level of physical activity or exercise also helps the doctor determine the cause of constipation.

Physical Examination. A physical exam may include a digital rectal exam with a gloved, lubricated finger to evaluate the tone of the muscle that closes off the anus (anal sphincter) and to detect tenderness, obstruction, or blood. In some cases, blood and thyroid tests may be necessary.

Extensive testing usually is reserved for people with severe symptoms, for those with sudden changes in number and consistency of bowel movements or blood in the stool, and for older adults. Because of an increased risk of colorectal cancer in older adults, the doctor may use these tests to rule out a diagnosis of cancer:

- Barium enema x-ray
- Sigmoidoscopy or colonoscopy
- Colorectal transit study
- Anorectal function tests.

Barium Enema X-Ray. A barium enema x-ray involves viewing the rectum, colon, and lower part of the small intestine to locate any problems. This part of the digestive tract is known as the bowel. This test may show intestinal obstruction and Hirschsprung's disease, a lack of nerves within the colon.

The night before the test, bowel cleansing, also called bowel prep, is necessary to clear the lower digestive tract. The patient drinks 8 ounces of a special liquid every 15 minutes for about 4 hours. This liquid flushes out the bowel. A clean bowel is important, because even a small amount of stool in the colon can hide details and result in an inaccurate exam.

Because the colon does not show up well on an x-ray, the doctor fills the organs with a barium enema, a chalky liquid to make the area visible. Once the mixture coats the organs, x-rays are taken that reveal their shape and condition. The patient may feel some abdominal cramping when the barium fills the colon, but usually feels little discomfort after the procedure. Stools may be a whitish color for a few days after the exam.

Sigmoidoscopy or Colonoscopy. An examination of the rectum and lower colon (sigmoid) is called a sigmoidoscopy. An examination of the rectum and entire colon is called a colonoscopy.

The night before a sigmoidoscopy, the patient usually has a liquid dinner and takes an enema at bedtime. A light breakfast and a cleansing enema an hour before the test may also be necessary.

To perform a sigmoidoscopy, the doctor uses a long, flexible tube with a light on the end called a sigmoidoscope to view the rectum and lower colon. First, the doctor examines the rectum with a gloved, lubricated finger. Then, the sigmoidoscope is inserted through the anus into the rectum and lower colon. The procedure may cause a mild sensation of wanting to move the bowels and abdominal pressure. Sometimes the doctor fills the organs with air to get a better view. The air may cause mild cramping.

To perform a colonoscopy, the doctor uses a flexible tube with a light on the end called a colonoscope to view the entire colon. This tube is longer than a sigmoidoscope. The same bowel cleansing used for the barium x-ray is needed to clear the bowel of waste. The patient is lightly sedated before the exam. During the exam, the patient lies on his or her side and the doctor inserts the tube through the anus and rectum into the colon. If an abnormality is seen, the doctor can use the colonoscope to remove a small piece of tissue for examination (biopsy). The patient may feel gassy and bloated after the procedure.

Colorectal Transit Study. This test, reserved for those with chronic constipation, shows how well food moves through the colon. The patient swallows capsules containing small markers, which are visible on x-ray. The movement of the markers through the colon is monitored with abdominal x-rays taken several times 3 to 7 days after the capsule is swallowed. The patient follows a high-fiber diet during the course of this test.

Anorectal Function Tests. These tests diagnose constipation caused by abnormal functioning of the anus or rectum (anorectal function). Anorectal manometry evaluates anal sphincter muscle function. A catheter or air-filled balloon inserted into the anus is slowly pulled back through the sphincter muscle to measure muscle tone and contractions.

Defecography is an x-ray of the anorectal area that evaluates completeness of stool elimination, identifies anorectal abnormalities, and evaluates rectal muscle contractions and relaxation. During the exam, the doctor fills the rectum with a soft paste that is the same consistency as stool. The patient sits on a toilet positioned inside an x-ray machine and then relaxes and squeezes the anus and expels the solution. The doctor studies the x-rays for anorectal problems that occurred while the patient emptied the paste.

How Is Constipation Treated?

Although treatment depends on the cause, severity, and duration, in most cases dietary and lifestyle changes will help relieve symptoms and help prevent constipation.

Diet. A diet with enough fiber (20 to 35 grams each day) helps form soft, bulky stool. A doctor or dietitian can help plan an appropriate diet. High-fiber foods include beans; whole grains and bran cereals; fresh fruits; and vegetables such as asparagus, brussels sprouts, cabbage, and carrots. For people prone to constipation, limiting foods that have little or no fiber such as ice cream, cheese, meat, and processed foods is also important.

Lifestyle Changes. Other changes that can help treat and prevent constipation include drinking enough water and other liquids such as fruit and vegetable juices and clear soup, engaging in daily exercise, and reserving enough time to have a bowel movement. In addition, the urge to have a bowel movement should not be ignored.

Laxatives. Most people who are mildly constipated do not need laxatives. However, for those who have made lifestyle changes and are still constipated, doctors may recommend laxatives or enemas for a limited time. These treatments can help retrain a chronically sluggish bowel. For children, short-term treatment with laxatives, along with retraining to establish regular bowel habits, also helps prevent constipation.

A doctor should determine when a patient needs a laxative and which form is best. Laxatives taken by mouth are available in liquid, tablet, gum, powder, and granule forms. They work in various ways:

- Bulk-forming laxatives generally are considered the safest but can interfere with absorption of some medicines. These laxatives, also known as fiber supplements, are taken with water. They absorb water in the intestine and make the stool softer. Brand names include Metamucil®, Citrucel®, and Serutan®.

- Stimulants cause rhythmic muscle contractions in the intestines. Brand names include Correctol®, Dulcolax®, Purge®, Feen-A-Mint®, and Senokot®. Studies suggest that phenolphthalein, an ingredient in some stimulant laxatives, might increase a person's risk for cancer. The Food and Drug Administration has proposed a ban on all over-the-counter products containing phenolphthalein. Most laxative makers have replaced or plan to replace phenolphthalein with a safer ingredient.

- Stool softeners provide moisture to the stool and prevent dehydration. These laxatives are often recommended after childbirth or surgery. Products include Colace®, Dialose®, and Surfak®.

- Lubricants grease the stool enabling it to move through the intestine more easily. Mineral oil is the most common lubricant.

- Saline laxatives act like a sponge to draw water into the colon for easier passage of stool. Laxatives in this group include Milk of Magnesia®, Citrate of Magnesia®, and Haley's M-O®.

People who are dependent on laxatives need to slowly stop using the medications. A doctor can assist in this process. In most people, this restores the colon's natural ability to contract.

Other Treatment. Treatment may be directed at a specific cause. For example, the doctor may recommend discontinuing medication or performing surgery to correct an anorectal problem such as rectal prolapse.

People with chronic constipation caused by anorectal dysfunction can use biofeedback to retrain the muscles that control release of bowel movements. Biofeedback involves using a sensor to monitor muscle activity that at the same time can be displayed on a computer screen allowing for an accurate assessment of body functions. A health care professional uses this information to help the patient learn how to use these muscles.

Surgical removal of the colon may be an option for people with severe symptoms caused by colonic inertia. However, the benefits of this surgery must be weighed against possible complications, which include abdominal pain and diarrhea.

Can Constipation Be Serious?

Sometimes constipation can lead to complications. These complications include hemorrhoids caused by straining to have a bowel movement or anal fissures (tears in the skin around the anus) caused when hard stool stretches the sphincter muscle. As a result, rectal bleeding may occur that appears as bright red streaks on the surface of the stool. Treatment for hemorrhoids may include warm tub baths, ice packs, and application of a cream to the affected area. Treatment for anal fissure may include stretching the sphincter muscle or surgical removal of tissue or skin in the affected area.

Sometimes straining causes a small amount of intestinal lining to push out from the anal opening. This condition is known as rectal prolapse and may lead to secretion of mucus from the anus. Usually, eliminating the cause of the prolapse such as straining or coughing is the only treatment necessary. Severe or chronic prolapse requires surgery to strengthen and tighten the anal sphincter muscle or to repair the prolapsed lining.

Constipation may also cause hard stool to pack the intestine and rectum so tightly that the normal pushing action of the colon is not enough to expel the stool. This condition, called fecal impaction, occurs most often in children and older adults. An impaction can be softened with mineral oil taken by mouth and an enema. After softening the impaction, the doctor may break up and remove part of the hardened stool by inserting one or two fingers in the anus.

Points to Remember

1. Constipation affects almost everyone at one time or another.

2. Many people think they are constipated when, in fact, their bowel movements are regular.

3. The most common causes of constipation are poor diet and lack of exercise.

4. Additional causes of constipation include medications, irritable bowel syndrome, abuse of laxatives, and specific diseases.

5. A medical history and physical examination may be the only diagnostic tests needed before the doctor suggests treatment.

6. In most cases, following these simple tips will help relieve symptoms and prevent recurrence of constipation:

   • Eat a well-balanced, high-fiber diet that includes beans, bran, whole grains, fresh fruits, and vegetables.
   • Drink plenty of liquids.
   • Exercise regularly.
   • Set aside time after breakfast or dinner for undisturbed visits to the toilet.
   • Do not ignore the urge to have a bowel movement.
   • Understand that normal bowel habits vary.
   • Whenever a significant or prolonged change in bowel habits occurs, check with a doctor.

7. Most people with mild constipation do not need laxatives. However, doctors may recommend laxatives for a limited time for people with chronic constipation.

Additional Resources

International Foundation for Functional Gastrointestinal Disorders
P.O. Box 17864
Milwaukee, WI 53217
(414) 964-1799

Intestinal Disease Foundation
1323 Forbes Avenue, Suite 200
Pittsburgh, PA 15219
(412) 261-5888

National Digestive Diseases Information Clearinghouse
2 Information Way
Bethesda, MD 20892-3570
E-mail: nddic@info.niddk.nih.gov

Chapter 15

Constipation in Children

Constipation means that bowel movements are hard and dry, difficult or painful to pass, and less frequent than usual. It is a common problem for children, but it is usually temporary and no cause for parents to be concerned.

When a child does not eat enough fiber, drink enough liquids, or get enough exercise, constipation is more likely to occur. It also happens when children ignore the urge to have a bowel movement, which they often do out of either embarrassment to use a public bathroom, fear or lack of confidence in the absence of a parent, or unwillingness to take a break from play. Sometimes constipation is caused by medicines or a disease.

Symptoms of constipation include:

- No bowel movement for several days or daily bowel movements that are hard and dry.
- Cramping abdominal pain.
- Nausea.
- Vomiting.
- Weight loss.
- Liquid or solid, clay-like stool in the child's underwear—a sign that stool is backed up in the rectum.

National Digestive Diseases Information Clearinghouse, National Institute of Diabetes and Digestive and Kidney Diseases (NIDDK), April 1998.

Constipation can make a bowel movement painful, so the child may try to prevent having one. Clenching buttocks, rocking up and down on toes, and turning red in the face are signs of trying to hold in a bowel movement.

Treatment depends on the child's age and the severity of the problem. Often eating more fiber (fruits, vegetables, whole-grain cereal), drinking more liquids, and getting more exercise solves the problem. Sometimes a child may need an enema to remove the stool or a laxative to soften it or prevent a future episode. However, laxatives can be dangerous to children and should only be given with a doctor's approval.

Although constipation is usually harmless, it can be a sign or cause of a more serious problem. A child should see a doctor if :

- Episodes of constipation last longer than 3 weeks.
- The child is unable to participate in normal activities.
- Small, painful tears appear in the skin around the anus.
- A small amount of the intestinal lining is pushed out of the anus (hemorrhoids).
- Normal pushing is not enough to expel stool.
- Liquid or soft stool leaks out of the anus.

Additional Information on Constipation in Children

The National Digestive Diseases Information Clearinghouse collects resource information on digestive diseases for the Combined Health Information Database (CHID). CHID is a database produced by health-related agencies of the Federal Government. This database provides titles, abstracts, and availability information for health information and health education resources.

You may access the CHID Online website and search CHID for the most up-to-date information on Constipation in Children.

Combined Health Information Database (CHID)
http://chid.nih.gov

Chapter 16

Crohn's Disease

Introduction

Crohn's disease causes inflammation in the small intestine. Crohn's disease usually occurs in the lower part of the small intestine, called the ileum, but it can affect any part of the digestive tract, from the mouth to the anus. The inflammation extends deep into the lining of the affected organ. The inflammation can cause pain and can make the intestines empty frequently, resulting in diarrhea.

Crohn's disease is an inflammatory bowel disease (IBD), the general name for diseases that cause inflammation in the intestines. Crohn's disease can be difficult to diagnose because its symptoms are similar to other intestinal disorders such as irritable bowel syndrome and to another type of IBD called ulcerative colitis. Ulcerative colitis causes inflammation and ulcers in the top layer of the lining of the large intestine.

Crohn's disease affects men and women equally and seems to run in some families. About 20 percent of people with Crohn's disease have a blood relative with some form of IBD, most often a brother or sister and sometimes a parent or child.

Crohn's disease may also be called ileitis or enteritis.

National Institute of Diabetes and Digestive and Kidney Diseases (NIDDK), NIH Pub. No. 98-4225, February 1998. The U.S. Government does not endorse or favor any specific commercial product or company. Brand names appearing in this text are used only because they are considered essential in the context of the information reported herein.

Questions and Answers about Crohn's Disease

What Causes Crohn's Disease?

Theories about what causes Crohn's disease abound, but none has been proven. The most popular theory is that the body's immune system reacts to a virus or a bacterium by causing ongoing inflammation in the intestine.

People with Crohn's disease tend to have abnormalities of the immune system, but doctors do not know whether these abnormalities are a cause or result of the disease. Crohn's disease is not caused by emotional distress.

What Are the Symptoms?

The most common symptoms of Crohn's disease are abdominal pain, often in the lower right area, and diarrhea. Rectal bleeding, weight loss, and fever may also occur. Bleeding may be serious and persistent, leading to anemia. Children with Crohn's disease may suffer delayed development and stunted growth.

How Is Crohn's Disease Diagnosed?

A thorough physical exam and a series of tests may be required to diagnose Crohn's disease.

Blood tests may be done to check for anemia, which could indicate bleeding in the intestines. Blood tests may also uncover a high white blood cell count, which is a sign of inflammation somewhere in the body. By testing a stool sample, the doctor can tell if there is bleeding or infection in the intestines.

The doctor may do an upper gastrointestinal (GI) series to look at the small intestine. For this test, the patient drinks barium, a chalky solution that coats the lining of the small intestine, before x-rays are taken. The barium shows up white on x-ray film, revealing inflammation or other abnormalities in the intestine.

The doctor may also do a colonoscopy. For this test, the doctor inserts an endoscope-a long, flexible, lighted tube linked to a computer and TV monitor-into the anus to see the inside of the large intestine. The doctor will be able to see any inflammation or bleeding. During the exam, the doctor may do a biopsy, which involves taking a sample of tissue from the lining of the intestine to view with a microscope.

If these tests show Crohn's disease, more x-rays of both the upper and lower digestive tract may be necessary to see how much is affected by the disease.

What Are the Complications of Crohn's Disease?

The most common complication is blockage of the intestine. Blockage occurs because the disease tends to thicken the intestinal wall with swelling and scar tissue, narrowing the passage. Crohn's disease may also cause sores, or ulcers, that tunnel through the affected area into surrounding tissues such as the bladder, vagina, or skin. The areas around the anus and rectum are often involved. The tunnels, called fistulas, are a common complication and often become infected. Sometimes fistulas can be treated with medicine, but in some cases they may require surgery.

Nutritional complications are common in Crohn's disease. Deficiencies of proteins, calories, and vitamins are well documented in Crohn's disease. These deficiencies may be caused by inadequate dietary intake, intestinal loss of protein, or poor absorption (malabsorption).

Other complications associated with Crohn's disease include arthritis, skin problems, inflammation in the eyes or mouth, kidney stones, gallstones, or other diseases of the liver and biliary system. Some of these problems resolve during treatment for disease in the digestive system, but some must be treated separately.

What Is the Treatment for Crohn's Disease?

Treatment for Crohn's disease depends on the location and severity of disease, complications, and response to previous treatment. The goals of treatment are to control inflammation, correct nutritional deficiencies, and relieve symptoms like abdominal pain, diarrhea, and rectal bleeding. Treatment may include drugs, nutrition supplements, surgery, or a combination of these options. At this time, treatment can help control the disease, but there is no cure.

Some people have long periods of remission, sometimes years, when they are free of symptoms. However, the disease usually recurs at various times over a person's lifetime. This changing pattern of the disease means one cannot always tell when a treatment has helped. Predicting when a remission may occur or when symptoms will return is not possible.

Someone with Crohn's disease may need medical care for a long time, with regular doctor visits to monitor the condition.

Drug Therapy. Most people are first treated with drugs containing mesalamine, a substance that helps control inflammation. Sulfasalazine is the most commonly used of these drugs. Patients who do not benefit from it or who cannot tolerate it may be put on other mesalamine-containing drugs, generally known as 5-ASA agents, such as Asacol, Dipentum, or Pentasa. Possible side effects of mesalamine preparations include nausea, vomiting, heartburn, diarrhea, and headache.

Some patients take corticosteroids to control inflammation. These drugs are the most effective for active Crohn's disease, but they can cause serious side effects, including greater susceptibility to infection.

Drugs that suppress the immune system are also used to treat Crohn's disease. Most commonly prescribed are 6-mercaptopurine and a related drug, azathioprine. Immunosuppressive agents work by blocking the immune reaction that contributes to inflammation. These drugs may cause side effects like nausea, vomiting, and diarrhea and may lower a person's resistance to infection. When patients are treated with a combination of corticosteroids and immunosuppressive drugs, the dose of corticosteriods can eventually be lowered. Some studies suggest that immunosuppressive drugs may enhance the effectiveness of corticosteroids.

The U.S. Food and Drug Administration has approved the drug infliximab (brand name, Remicade) for the treatment of moderate to severe Crohn's disease that does not respond to standard therapies (mesalamine substances, corticosteroids, immunosuppressive agents) and for the treatment of open, draining fistulas. Infliximab, the first treatment approved specifically for Crohn's disease, is an anti-tumor necrosis factor (TNF) substance. TNF is a protein produced by the immune system that may cause the inflammation associated with Crohn's disease. Anti-TNF removes TNF from the bloodstream before it reaches the intestines, thereby preventing inflammation. Investigators will continue to study patients taking infliximab to determine its long-term safety and efficacy.

Antibiotics are used to treat bacterial overgrowth in the small intestine caused by stricture, fistulas, or prior surgery. For this common problem, the doctor may prescribe one or more of the following antibiotics: ampicillin, sulfonamide, cephalosporin, tetracycline, or metronidazole.

Diarrhea and crampy abdominal pain are often relieved when the inflammation subsides, but additional medication may also be necessary. Several antidiarrheal agents could be used, including diphenoxylate, loperamide, and codeine. Patients who are dehydrated because of diarrhea will be treated with fluids and electrolytes.

Nutrition Supplementation. The doctor may recommend nutritional supplements, especially for children whose growth has been slowed. Special high-calorie liquid formulas are sometimes used for this purpose. A small number of patients may need periods of feeding by vein. This can help patients who need extra nutrition temporarily, those whose intestines need to rest, or those whose intestines cannot absorb enough nutrition from food.

Surgery. Surgery to remove part of the intestine can help Crohn's disease but cannot cure it. The inflammation tends to return next to the area of intestine that has been removed. Many Crohn's disease patients require surgery, either to relieve symptoms that do not respond to medical therapy or to correct complications such as blockage, perforation, abscess, or bleeding in the intestine.

Some people who have Crohn's disease in the large intestine need to have their entire colon removed in an operation called colectomy. A small opening is made in the front of the abdominal wall, and the tip of the ileum is brought to the skin's surface. This opening, called a stoma, is where waste exits the body. The stoma is about the size of a quarter and is usually located in the right lower part of the abdomen near the beltline. A pouch is worn over the opening to collect waste, and the patient empties the pouch as needed. The majority of colectomy patients go on to live normal, active lives.

Sometimes only the diseased section of intestine is removed and no stoma is needed. In this operation, the intestine is cut above and below the diseased area and reconnected.

Because Crohn's disease often recurs after surgery, people considering it should carefully weigh its benefits and risks compared with other treatments. Surgery may not be appropriate for everyone. People faced with this decision should get as much information as possible from doctors, nurses who work with colon surgery patients (enterostomal therapists), and other patients. Patient advocacy organizations can suggest support groups and other information resources. (See Resources for the names of such organizations.)

People with Crohn's disease may feel well and be free of symptoms for substantial spans of time when their disease is not active. Despite the need to take medication for long periods of time and occasional hospitalizations, most people with Crohn's disease are able to hold jobs, raise families, and function successfully at home and in society.

Research

Researchers continue to look for more effective treatments. Examples of investigational treatments include

Anti-TNF. Research has shown that cells affected by Crohn's disease contain a cytokine, a protein produced by the immune system, called tumor necrosis factor (TNF). TNF may be responsible for the inflammation of Crohn's disease. Anti-TNF is a substance that finds TNF in the bloodstream, binds to it, and removes it before it can reach the intestines and cause inflammation. In studies, anti-TNF seems particularly helpful in closing fistulas.

Interleukin 10. Interleukin 10 (IL-10) is a cytokine that suppresses inflammation. Researchers are now studying the effectiveness of synthetic IL-10 in treating Crohn's disease.

Antibiotics. Antibiotics are now used to treat the bacterial infections that often accompany Crohn's disease, but some research suggests that they might also be useful as a primary treatment for active Crohn's disease.

Budesonide. Researchers recently identified a new corticosteroid called budesonide that appears to be as effective as other corticosteroids but causes fewer side effects.

Methotrexate and cyclosporine. These are immunosuppressive drugs that may be useful in treating Crohn's disease. One potential benefit of methotrexate and cyclosporine is that they appear to work faster than traditional immunosuppressive drugs.

Zinc. Free radicals-molecules produced during fat metabolism, stress, and infection, among other things-may contribute to inflammation in Crohn's disease. Free radicals sometimes cause cell damage when they interact with other molecules in the body. The mineral zinc removes free radicals from the bloodstream. Studies are under way to determine whether zinc supplementation might reduce inflammation.

Can Diet Control Crohn's Disease?

No special diet has been proven effective for preventing or treating this disease. Some people find their symptoms are made worse by milk, alcohol, hot spices, or fiber. People are encouraged to follow a nutritious diet and avoid any foods that seem to worsen symptoms. But there are no consistent rules.

People should take vitamin supplements only on their doctor's advice.

Is Pregnancy Safe for Women with Crohn's Disease?

Research has shown that the course of pregnancy and delivery is usually not impaired in women with Crohn's disease. Even so, women with Crohn's disease should discuss the matter with their doctors before pregnancy. Most children born to women with Crohn's disease are unaffected. Children who do get the disease are sometimes more severely affected than adults, with slowed growth and delayed sexual development in some cases.

Resources

Crohn's & Colitis Foundation of America, Inc.
386 Park Avenue South, 17th Floor
New York, NY 10016-8804
Tel: (800) 932-2423 or (212) 685-3440
E-mail: info@ccfa.org
Home Page: http://www.ccfa.org/

Pediatric Crohn's & Colitis Association, Inc.
P.O. Box 188
Newton, MA 02468
Tel: (617) 489-5854
E-mail: questions@pcca.hypermart.net
Home Page: http://pcca.hypermart.net

Pull-thru Network
4 Woody Lane
Westport, CT 06880
Tel: (203) 221-7530
E-mail: pullthrunw@aol.com
Home page: http://members.aol.com/pullthrunw/Pullthru.html

Reach Out for Youth with Ileitis and Colitis, Inc.
15 Chemung Place
Jericho, NY 11753
Tel: (516) 822-8010

United Ostomy Association
36 Executive Park, Suite 120
Irvine, CA 92714
Tel: (800) 826-0826 or (714) 660-8624
E-mail: uoa@deltanet.com
Home Page: http://www.uoa.org/

Chapter 17

Cyclic Vomiting Syndrome

What Is Cyclic Vomiting Syndrome?

CVS is an uncommon, unexplained disorder of children and some adults that was first described by Dr. S. Gee in 1882. The condition is characterized by recurrent, prolonged attacks of severe nausea, vomiting and prostration with no apparent cause. Vomiting occurs at frequent intervals (5-10 times an hour at the peak) for hours to 10 days (1-4 most common). The episodes tend to be similar to each other in symptoms and duration and are self-limited. The person is typically well between episodes.

Occurrence

The onset of CVS occurs in infancy through adulthood but most commonly between the ages of 3 and 7. It can persist for months to decades. The episode may recur several times a year or several times a month. Females are affected slightly more than males. The person may be prone to motion sickness, and there is often a family history of migraine.

Symptoms

Episodes may begin at any time, but typically start during the night or early morning. There is relentless nausea with repeated bouts of vomiting or retching. The person is very pale and resists talking. They often drool or spit and have an extreme thirst. There is often intense abdominal pain and less often headache, low-grade fever and diarrhea. Prolonged vomiting may cause mild bleeding from irritation of the esophagus. Patients are described as being in a "conscious coma." The symptoms are frightening to the person and family and can be life-threatening due to dehydration and electrolyte imbalance.

Diagnosis

CVS has been difficult to diagnose because it is infrequently seen in clinical practice and because vomiting may be caused by a large number of common disorders other than CVS. There are as yet no blood tests, x-rays or other specific procedures used to diagnose the disorder. The diagnosis is made by careful review of the patient's history, physical examination, and studies to rule out other diseases that may cause vomiting similar to that seen in people with CVS.

Triggers

Although some patients know of nothing that triggers attacks, many can identify specific circumstances that seem to bring on their episodes. Colds, flus and other infections, emotional stress, and intense excitement (birthdays, holidays, vacations) are the most frequently reported triggers. Specific foods or anesthetics may also play a role.

Related Terms

- abdominal migraine
- bilious attacks
- periodic syndrome
- recurrent vomiting

Treatment

Treatment is generally supportive with early intervention in a dark quiet environment for sleep and IV fluids when needed. Medication trials sometimes succeed in finding something to prevent, shorten, or abort the episodes. An essential component of treatment is the doctor-patient-family relationship. It involves a physician who does his/her best to understand CVS, is supportive and willing to coordinate the care in collaboration with all involved. A family/professional network, such as Cyclic Vomiting Syndrome Association (CVSA), can help heal a family that has been in doubt and despair for years.

References

Abu-Arafeh, I. and Russell, G. (1995). "Cyclical vomiting syndrome in children: A population based study," *Journal of Pediatric Gastroenterology and Nutrition*, 21(4), 254-258.

Abu-Arafeh, I. and Russell, G. (1995). "Prevalence and clinical features of abdominal migraine compared with those of migraine headache," *Archives of Disease in Childhood*, 72(5), 413-7.

Anderson, J., Lockhart, J., Sugerman, K., Weinberg, W. (1997). "Effective prophylactic therapy for cyclic vomiting syndrome in children using amitriptyline or cyproheptadine," *Pediatrics*, 100(6), 977-981.

Boles, R. G., Chun, N., Dcnadheera, D., Wong, L.-J.C. (1997). "Cyclic vomiting syndrome and mitochondrial DNA mutations," *Lancet*, 350, 1299-1300.

Fleisher, D.R. and Matar, M. (1993). The cyclic vomiting syndrome: A report of 71 cases and literature review. *Journal of Pediatric Gastroenterology and Nutrition*, 17(4), 361-369.

Fleisher, D.R. (1994). "Cyclic vomiting." In P.E. Hyman & C. DiLorenzo (Eds.), *Pediatric Gastrointestinal Motility Disorders*, (pp. 89-103). New York: Academy Professional Information Services.

Fleisher, D.R. (1997). "Cyclic vomiting syndrome: A paroxysmal disorder of brain-gut interaction," *Journal of Pediatric Gastroenterology and Nutrition*, 25, Supplement 1, S13-15.

Forbes, D. (1995). "Cyclical Vomiting Syndrome," *Journal of Paediatric Child Health*, 31, 67-69.

Gee, S. (1882). "On fitful or recurrent vomiting," *Saint Bartholomew's Hospital Reports*, 18, 1-6.

Hoyt and Stickler (1960). "A study of 44 children with the syndrome of recurrent vomiting," *Pediatrics*, 25, 775-780.

Hyman, P.E. and Fleisher, D.R. (1997). "Pediatric functional gastrointestinal disorders," *Journal of Pediatric Gastroenterology and Nutrition*, 25, Supplement 1, S11-12.

Lee, M. and Feldman, M. (1997). "Cyclic vomiting syndrome." In M. Sleisenger, J. Fordtran, M. Feldman, B. Scharschmidt (Eds.) *Gastrointestinal Disease, 6th edition,* volume 1, (p.1 21). Philadelphia: Saunders.

Li, B U.K. (1996). "Cyclic vomiting: New understanding of an old disorder," *Contemporary Pediatrics*, 13(7), 48-62.

Li, B U.K. (Ed.) (1995). "Cyclical vomiting syndrome: Proceedings of the international scientific symposium on cyclic vomiting syndrome held at St. Bartholomew's Hospital, London, England, July 29-30, 1994," *Journal of Pediatric Gastroenterology and Nutrition*, 21 (Suppl.1).

Li, B U.K., et al. (In press). Is cyclic vomiting related to migraine? *Journal of Pediatrics*.

Li, B U.K., Sarna, S. Issenman, R. (Eds.) (in press). "Proceedings of the Second Scientific Symposium on CVS Held at the Medical College of Wisconsin, USA, April 17 - 18, 1998," *Digestive Diseases and Sciences*.

Olness, K., Stein, M.T., Katz, R. M., Jellinek. M.S. (1997). Challenging case—cyclic vomiting. *Developmental and Behavioral Pediatrics*, 18(4), 267-270.

Pfau, B.T., Li, B U.K., et al. (1996). "Differentiating cyclic from chronic vomiting patterns in children," *Pediatrics*, 97, 364-368.

Symon, D.N.K. and Russell, G. (1986). "Abdominal migraine: A childhood syndrome defined," *Cephalalgia*, 6, 223-8.

Symon, D.N.K. and Russell, G. (1995). "The relationship between cyclic vomiting syndrome and abdominal migraine." In B U.K. Li (Ed.) Cyclical vomiting syndrome: Proceedings of the international scientific symposium on cyclic vomiting syndrome held at St. Bartholomew's Hospital, London, England, July 29-30, 1994. *Journal of Pediatric Gastroenterology and Nutrition*, 21 (Suppl. 1)

Withers, G.D., Silburn, S.R., Forbes, D.A. (1998). "Cyclic vomiting syndrome: a descriptive analysis of symptoms, precipitants, aetiology and treatment," *Acta Paediatrica*, 87, 272-277.

For More Information

Cyclic Vomiting Syndrome Association
13180 Caroline Court
Elm Grove, WI 53122
Telephone (414) 784-6842
Fax (414) 821-5494
E-mail kadams@post.its.mcw.edu
Internet CVS information: http://www.beaker.iupui.edu/cvsa

Chapter 18

Diarrhea

Quesions about Diarrhea

What Is Diarrhea?

Diarrhea—loose, watery stools occurring more than three times in one day—is a common problem that usually lasts a day or two and goes away on its own without any special treatment. However, prolonged diarrhea can be a sign of other problems.

Diarrhea can cause dehydration, which means the body lacks enough fluid to function properly. Dehydration is particularly dangerous in children and the elderly, and it must be treated promptly to avoid serious health problems. Dehydration is discussed below.

People of all ages can get diarrhea. The average adult has a bout of diarrhea about four times a year.

What Causes Diarrhea?

Diarrhea may be caused by a temporary problem, like an infection, or a chronic problem, like an intestinal disease. A few of the more common causes of diarrhea are:

This chapter contains text from "Diarrhea," National Institute of Diabetes and Digestive and Kidney Diseases (NIDDK), NIH Pub. No. 99-2749, January 1999; and "Tips for Controlling Diarrhea," Intestinal Disease Foundation, Inc., 1323 Forbes Ave., Suite 200, Pittsburgh, PA 15219, (412) 261-5888; reprinted with permission.

- *Bacterial infections.* Several types of bacteria, consumed through contaminated food or water, can cause diarrhea. Common culprits include Campylobacter, Salmonella, Shigella, and Escherichia coli.

- *Viral infections.* Many viruses cause diarrhea, including rotavirus, Norwalk virus, cytomegalovirus, herpes simplex virus, and viral hepatitis.

- *Food intolerances.* Some people are unable to digest a component of food, such as lactose, the sugar found in milk.

- *Parasites.* Parasites can enter the body through food or water and settle in the digestive system. Parasites that cause diarrhea include Giardia lamblia, Entamoeba histolytica, and Cryptosporidium.

- *Reaction to medicines,* such as antibiotics, blood pressure medications, and antacids containing magnesium.

- *Intestinal diseases,* like inflammatory bowel disease or celiac disease.

- *Functional bowel disorders,* such as irritable bowel syndrome, in which the intestines do not work normally.

Some people develop diarrhea after stomach surgery or removal of the gallbladder. The reason may be a change in how quickly food moves through the digestive system after stomach surgery or an increase in bile in the colon that can occur after gallbladder surgery.

In many cases, the cause of diarrhea cannot be found. As long as diarrhea goes away on its own, an extensive search for the cause is not usually necessary.

People who visit foreign countries are at risk for traveler's diarrhea, which is caused by eating food or drinking water contaminated with bacteria, viruses, or, sometimes, parasites. Traveler's diarrhea is a particular problem for people visiting developing countries. Visitors to the United States, Canada, most European countries, Japan, Australia, and New Zealand do not face much risk for traveler's diarrhea.

What Are the Symptoms?

Diarrhea may be accompanied by cramping abdominal pain, bloating, nausea, or an urgent need to use the bathroom. Depending on the cause, a person may have a fever or bloody stools.

Diarrhea can be either acute or chronic. The acute form, which lasts less than 3 weeks, is usually related to a bacterial, viral, or parasitic infection. Chronic diarrhea lasts more than 3 weeks and is usually related to functional disorders like irritable bowel syndrome or diseases like celiac disease or inflammatory bowel disease.

Diarrhea in Children

Children can have acute (short-term) or chronic (long-term) forms of diarrhea. Causes include bacteria, viruses, parasites, medications, functional disorders, and food sensitivities. Infection with the rotavirus is the most common cause of acute childhood diarrhea. Rotavirus diarrhea usually resolves in 5 to 8 days. A vaccine to prevent rotavirus infection is now available for infants under 6 months of age.

Medications to treat diarrhea in adults can be dangerous to children and should be given only under a doctor's guidance.

Diarrhea can be dangerous in newborns and infants. In small children, severe diarrhea lasting just a day or two can lead to dehydration. Because a child can die from dehydration within a few days, the main treatment for diarrhea in children is rehydration. Rehydration is discussed below.

Take your child to the doctor if any of the following symptoms appear:

- Stools containing blood or pus, or black stools.
- Temperature above 101.4 degrees Fahrenheit.
- No improvement after 24 hours.
- Signs of dehydration (see below).

What Is Dehydration?

General signs of dehydration include:

- Thirst.
- Less frequent urination.
- Dry skin.
- Fatigue.
- Light-headedness.

Signs of dehydration in children include:

- Dry mouth and tongue.
- No tears when crying.

- No wet diapers for 3 hours or more.
- Sunken abdomen, eyes, or cheeks.
- High fever.
- Listlessness or irritability.
- Skin that does not flatten when pinched and released.

If you suspect that you or your child is dehydrated, call the doctor immediately. Severe dehydration may require hospitalization.

When Should a Doctor Be Consulted?

Although usually not harmful, diarrhea can become dangerous or signal a more serious problem. You should see the doctor if:

- You have diarrhea for more than 3 days.
- You have severe pain in the abdomen or rectum.
- You have a fever of 102 degrees Fahrenheit or higher.
- You see blood in your stool or have black, tarry stools.
- You have signs of dehydration.

If your child has diarrhea, do not hesitate to call the doctor for advice. Diarrhea can be dangerous in children if too much fluid is lost and not replaced quickly.

What Tests Might the Doctor Do?

Diagnostic tests to find the cause of diarrhea include the following:

- *Medical history and physical examination.* The doctor will need to know about your eating habits and medication use and will examine you for signs of illness.

- *Stool culture.* Lab technicians analyze a sample of stool to check for bacteria, parasites, or other signs of disease or infection.

- *Blood tests.* Blood tests can be helpful in ruling out certain diseases.

- *Fasting tests.* To find out if a food intolerance or allergy is causing the diarrhea, the doctor may ask you to avoid lactose (found in milk products), carbohydrates, wheat, or other foods to see whether the diarrhea responds to a change in diet.

- *Sigmoidoscopy*. For this test, the doctor uses a special instrument to look at the inside of the rectum and lower part of the colon.

- *Colonoscopy*. This test is similar to sigmoidoscopy, but the doctor looks at the entire colon.

What Is the Treatment?

In most cases, replacing lost fluid to prevent dehydration is the only treatment necessary. (See "Preventing Dehydration" below.) Medicines that stop diarrhea may be helpful in some cases, but they are not recommended for people whose diarrhea is from a bacterial infection or parasite—stopping the diarrhea traps the organism in the intestines, prolonging the problem. Instead, doctors usually prescribe antibiotics. Viral causes are either treated with medication or left to run their course, depending on the severity and type of the virus.

Preventing Dehydration. Dehydration occurs when the body has lost too much fluid and electrolytes (the salts potassium and sodium). The fluid and electrolytes lost during diarrhea need to be replaced promptly—the body cannot function properly without them. Dehydration is particularly dangerous for children, who can die from it within a matter of days.

Although water is extremely important in preventing dehydration, it does not contain electrolytes. To maintain electrolyte levels, you should also have chicken or beef broth, which contains sodium, and fruit and cola drinks, which contain potassium.

For children, doctors often recommend a special rehydration solution that contains the nutrients they need. You can buy this solution in the grocery store without a prescription. Examples include Pedialyte, Ceralyte, and Infalyte. (The U.S. Government does not endorse or favor any specific commercial product or company. Brand names appearing in this text are used only because they are considered essential in the context of the information.)

Tips About Food. Until diarrhea subsides, try to avoid milk products and foods that are greasy, high-fiber, or very sweet. These foods tend to aggravate diarrhea.

As you improve, you can add soft, bland foods to your diet, including bananas, plain rice, boiled potatoes, toast, crackers, cooked carrots, and baked chicken without the skin or fat. For children, the pediatrician may recommend what is called the BRAT diet: bananas, rice, applesauce, and toast.

Preventing Traveler's Diarrhea

Traveler's diarrhea happens when you consume food or water contaminated with bacteria, viruses, or parasites. You can take the following precautions to prevent traveler's diarrhea when you go abroad:

- Do not drink any tap water, not even when brushing your teeth.
- Do not drink unpasteurized milk or dairy products.
- Do not use ice made from tap water.
- Avoid all raw fruits and vegetables (including lettuce and fruit salad) unless they can be peeled and you peel them yourself.
- Do not eat raw or rare meat and fish.
- Do not eat meat or shellfish that is not hot when served to you.
- Do not eat food from street vendors.

You can safely drink bottled water (if you are the one to break the seal), carbonated soft drinks, and hot drinks like coffee or tea.

Depending on where you are going and how long you are staying, your doctor may recommend that you take antibiotics before leaving to protect you from possible infection.

Points to Remember

- Diarrhea is a common problem that usually resolves on its own.

- Diarrhea is dangerous if a person becomes dehydrated.

- Causes include viral, bacterial, or parasitic infections; food intolerance; reactions to medicine; intestinal diseases; and functional bowel disorders.

- Treatment involves replacing lost fluids and electrolytes. Depending on the cause of the problem, a person might also need medication to stop the diarrhea or treat an infection. Children may need an oral rehydration solution to replace lost fluids and electrolytes.

- Call the doctor if a person with diarrhea has severe pain in the abdomen or rectum, a fever of 102 degrees Fahrenheit or higher, blood in the stool, signs of dehydration, or diarrhea for more than 3 days.

Tips for Controlling Diarrhea

How to Help Control Diarrhea

Diet. Diarrhea may be controlled to some extent through diet. Certain foods produce loose stools and should be avoided if diarrhea is a problem.

Eating behaviors. The number of meals, mealtime circumstances, and even food temperature can help alleviate diarrhea.

Please note. If you have problems with diarrhea, don't cut out all the following foods at once. It is very important not to cut out foods unnecessarily, since malnutrition may result.

When to call your doctor. Diarrhea can be caused by many things. A doctor should be overseeing your care if your diarrhea lasts more than a few days.

Choose Foods That "Bind"

Certain foods that are high in soluble fiber delay the emptying of the stomach. By choosing a binding food at mealtime you will be helping to slow down your gastrointestinal tract. These are "safe" foods.

- applesauce
- carrots
- grated apples
- green beans
- potatoes
- barley
- oats/oat bran
- boiled white rice
- avocados
- tapioca
- smooth peanut butter
- Metamucil or other fiber supplement

Beverage Choices

Best beverage choices:

- broths
- nectars (like peach or apricot)

- nonacidic juices
- Gatorade

Avoid caffeine, beer and red wine—they're all gastrointestinal stimulants.

Eating and Drinking Behaviors

- Eat smaller portions.
- Avoid extremely hot meals—they tend to increase intestinal activity.
- Consume a lot of liquids, but in the following way:
  - Minimize liquid intake at mealtime, and drink fluids between meals.
  - Drink liquids at room temperatures.
- Don't skip meals.
- Practice being very calm at meal time, consciously relaxing during the meal and when you start to feel the urge to go. When your system is accustomed to frequent diarrhea, it can develop a reflexive action that operates independently of what you are eating. You may be able to break this reflex by conscious relaxation.

Foods to Avoid

- Avoid gas-forming foods
- Try limiting or eliminating dairy products
- Try limiting or eliminating some of the following:
  - baked beans
  - onions
  - broccoli
  - chocolate
  - prune juice
  - nuts
  - raw vegetables
  - fructose
  - excessive coffee
  - licorice
  - corn
  - raw fruits
  - spinach
  - large meals

- dried beans
- cauliflower
- whole grains
- garlic
- greasy, fatty food
- sugar
- shellfish
- Nutrasweet
- Sorbitol/Mannitol
- MSG
- processed meats
- heavily spiced foods
- hot beverages/soups

Don't Forget the Potassium!

Since diarrhea may deplete the body of electrolytes, make sure that you consume high potassium foods. Some good choices include:

- apricot or peach nectars
- nectarines
- fish
- avocado
- boiled or mashed potatoes
- bananas (if tolerated)

Other Tips

- Use an Imodium AD type product (liquid works faster) as soon as you realize you have a problem—take the full dose allowed right from the beginning. You can even take it before going out, to avoid a problem.

- Mix one teaspoon of Sure-jell (found in the supermarket with supplies for preserving food) with one quarter cup non-citrus juice and drink 30 minutes before eating.

For More Information

The Intestinal Disease Foundation is a network of people with chronic intestinal illnesses, reaching out to help others in the same situation, with educational and support activities. For further information, call IDF at (412) 261-5888.

Chapter 19

Diverticulosis and Diverticulitis

Introduction

Most people have in their colons small pouches that bulge outward through weak spots, like an inner tube that pokes through weak places in a tire. Each pouch is called a diverticulum. Pouches are diverticula. The condition of having diverticula is called diverticulosis. About half of all Americans age 60 to 80, and almost everyone over age 80, have diverticulosis.

When the pouches become infected or inflamed, the condition is called diverticulitis. This happens in 10 to 25 percent of people with diverticulosis. Diverticulosis and diverticulitis are also called *diverticular disease*.

Questions and Answers about Diverticulosis and Diverticulitis

What Causes Diverticular Disease?

Doctors believe a low-fiber diet is the main cause of diverticular disease. The disease was first noticed in the United States in the early 1900's. At about the same time, processed foods were introduced to the American diet. Many processed foods contain refined, low-fiber flour. Unlike whole-wheat flour, refined flour has no wheat bran.

National Institute of Diabetes and Digestive and Kidney Diseases (NIDDK), NIH Publication No. 97-1163, updated November 1998.

137

Diverticular disease is common in developed or industrialized countries—particularly the United States, England, and Australia—where low-fiber diets are common. The disease is rare in countries of Asia and Africa, where people eat high-fiber vegetable diets.

Fiber is the part of fruits, vegetables, and grains that the body cannot digest. Some fiber dissolves easily in water (soluble fiber). It takes on a soft, jelly-like texture in the intestines. Some fiber passes almost unchanged through the intestines (insoluble fiber). Both kinds of fiber help make stools soft and easy to pass. Fiber also prevents constipation.

Constipation makes the muscles strain to move stool that is too hard. It is the main cause of increased pressure in the colon. The excess pressure causes the weak spots in the colon to bulge out and become diverticula.

Diverticulitis occurs when diverticula become infected or inflamed. Doctors are not certain what causes the infection. It may begin when

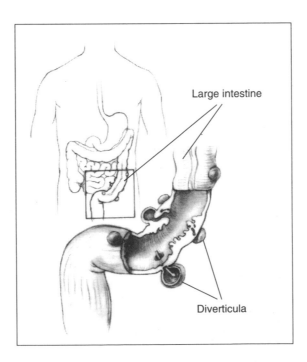

Figure 19.1. Diverticula are bulging pouches in the colon.

stool or bacteria are caught in the diverticula. An attack of diverticulitis can develop suddenly and without warning.

What Are the Symptoms?

Diverticulosis. Most people with diverticulosis do not have any discomfort or symptoms. However, symptoms may include mild cramps, bloating, and constipation. Other diseases such as irritable bowel syndrome (IBS) and stomach ulcers cause similar problems, so these symptoms do not always mean a person has diverticulosis. You should visit your doctor if you have these troubling symptoms.

Diverticulitis. The most common symptom of diverticulitis is abdominal pain. The most common sign is tenderness around the left side of the lower abdomen. If infection is the cause, fever, nausea, vomiting, chills, cramping, and constipation may occur as well. The severity of symptoms depends on the extent of the infection and complications.

Are There Complications?

Diverticulitis can lead to complications such as infections, perforations or tears, blockages, or bleeding. These complications always require treatment to prevent them from progressing and causing serious illness.

Bleeding. Bleeding from diverticula is a rare complication. When diverticula bleed, blood may appear in the toilet or in your stool. Bleeding can be severe, but it may stop by itself and not require treatment. Doctors believe bleeding diverticula are caused by a small blood vessel in a diverticulum that weakens and finally bursts. If you have bleeding from the rectum, you should see your doctor. If the bleeding does not stop, surgery may be necessary.

Abscess, Perforation, and Peritonitis. The infection causing diverticulitis often clears up after a few days of treatment with antibiotics. If the condition gets worse, an abscess may form in the colon.

An abscess is an infected area with pus that may cause swelling and destroy tissue. Sometimes, the infected diverticula may develop small holes, called perforations. These perforations allow pus to leak out of the colon into the abdominal area. If the abscess is small and remains in the colon, it may clear up after treatment with antibiotics. If the abscess does not clear up with antibiotics, the doctor may need to drain it.

To drain the abscess, the doctor uses a needle and a small tube called a catheter. The doctor inserts the needle through the skin and drains the fluid through the catheter. This procedure is called "percutaneous catheter drainage." Sometimes surgery is needed to clean the abscess and, if necessary, remove part of the colon.

A large abscess can become a serious problem if the infection leaks out and contaminates areas outside the colon. Infection that spreads into the abdominal cavity is called peritonitis. Peritonitis requires immediate surgery to clean the abdominal cavity and remove the damaged part of the colon. Without surgery, peritonitis can be fatal.

Fistula. A fistula is an abnormal connection of tissue between two organs or between an organ and the skin. When damaged tissues come into contact with each other during infection, they sometimes stick together. If they heal that way, a fistula forms. When diverticulitis-related infection spreads outside the colon, the colon's tissue may stick to nearby tissues. The most common organs involved are the urinary bladder, small intestine, and skin.

The most common type of fistula occurs between the bladder and the colon. It affects men more than women. This type of fistula can result in a severe, long-lasting infection of the urinary tract. The problem can be corrected with surgery to remove the fistula and the affected part of the colon.

Intestinal Obstruction. The scarring caused by infection may cause partial or total blockage of the large intestine. When this happens, the colon is unable to move bowel contents normally. When the obstruction totally blocks the intestine, emergency surgery is necessary. Partial blockage is not an emergency, so the surgery to correct it can be planned.

How Does the Doctor Diagnose Diverticular Disease?

To diagnose diverticular disease, the doctor asks about medical history, does a physical exam, and may perform one or more diagnostic tests. Because most people do not have symptoms, diverticulosis is often found through tests ordered for another ailment.

Medical History and Physical Exam. When taking a medical history, the doctor may ask about bowel habits, symptoms, pain, diet, and medications. The physical exam usually involves a digital rectal exam. To perform this test, the doctor inserts a gloved, lubricated finger into the rectum to detect tenderness, blockage, or blood. The doctor may check stool for signs of bleeding and test blood for signs of infection. The doctor may also order x-rays or other tests.

What Is the Treatment for Diverticular Disease?

A high-fiber diet and, occasionally, mild pain medications will help relieve symptoms in most cases. Sometimes an attack of diverticulitis is serious enough to require a hospital stay and possibly surgery.

Diverticulosis. Increasing the amount of fiber in the diet may reduce symptoms of diverticulosis and prevent complications such as diverticulitis. Fiber keeps stool soft and lowers pressure inside the colon so that bowel contents can move through easily. The American Dietetic Association recommends 20 to 35 grams of fiber each day. Table 19.1 shows the amount of fiber in several foods that you can easily add to your diet.

The doctor may also recommend drinking a fiber product such as Citrucel or Metamucil once a day. These products are mixed with water and provide about 4 to 6 grams of fiber for an 8-ounce glass.

Until recently, many doctors suggested avoiding foods with small seeds such as tomatoes or strawberries because they believed that particles could lodge in the diverticula and cause inflammation. However, this is now a controversial point and no evidence supports this recommendation.

If cramps, bloating, and constipation are problems, the doctor may prescribe a short course of pain medication. However, many medications affect emptying of the colon, an undesirable side effect for people with diverticulosis.

Diverticulitis. Treatment for diverticulitis focuses on clearing up the infection and inflammation, resting the colon, and preventing or minimizing complications. An attack of diverticulitis without complications may respond to antibiotics within a few days if treated early.

To help the colon rest, the doctor may recommend bed rest and a liquid diet, along with a pain reliever or a drug such as propantheline (Pro-Banthine) to control muscle spasms in the colon.

An acute attack with severe pain or severe infection may require a hospital stay. Most acute cases of diverticulitis are treated with antibiotics and a liquid diet. The antibiotics are given by injection into a vein. In some cases, however, surgery may be necessary.

Table 19. 1. Amount of Fiber in Some Foods

Fruits

raspberries	1 cup	=	6 grams of fiber
apple	1	=	3 grams
tangerine	1	=	2 grams
peach	1	=	1 gram

Vegetables

acorn squash	3/4 cup	=	4 grams
brussels sprouts	1/2 cup	=	3 grams
cabbage	1/2 cup	=	2 grams
carrot	1	=	2 grams
potato, peeled	1	=	2 grams
tomato	1	=	2 grams
asparagus	1/2 cup	=	1 gram
broccoli	1/2 cup	=	1 gram
cauliflower	1/2 cup	=	1 gram
romaine lettuce	1 cup	=	1 gram
spinach	1/2 cup	=	1 gram
zucchini	1 cup	=	1 gram

Starchy Vegetables

black-eyed peas	1/2 cup	=	4 grams
lima beans	1/2 cup	=	4 grams
kidney beans	1/2 cup	=	3 grams

Grains

brown rice	1 cup	=	3 grams
oatmeal	2/3 cup	=	3 grams
whole-wheat cereal	1 cup	=	3 grams
whole-wheat bread	1 slice	=	2 grams
white rice	1 cup	=	1 gram

Source: JAT Pennington. *Sixteenth Edition of Bowes and Church's Food Values of Portions Commonly Used.* J.B. Lippincott Publishing Co., Philadelphia, PA. 1994.

When Is Surgery Necessary?

If attacks are severe or frequent, the doctor may advise surgery. The surgeon opens the abdomen and removes the affected part of the colon. The remaining sections of the colon are rejoined. This type of surgery, called colon resection, aims to keep attacks from coming back and to prevent complications. The doctor may also recommend surgery for complications of a fistula or intestinal obstruction.

If antibiotics do not correct the attack, emergency surgery may be required. Other reasons for emergency surgery include a large abscess, perforation, peritonitis, or continued bleeding.

Emergency surgery usually involves two operations. The first surgery will clear the infected abdominal cavity and remove part of the colon. Because of infection and sometimes obstruction, it is not safe to rejoin the colon during the first operation. The surgeon creates a temporary hole, or stoma, in the abdomen during the first operation. The end of the colon is connected to the hole, a procedure called a colostomy, to allow normal eating and bowel movement. The stool goes into a bag attached to the opening in the abdomen. In the second operation, the surgeon rejoins the ends of the colon.

Points to Remember

1. Diverticulosis occurs when small pouches, called diverticula, bulge outward through weak spots in the colon (large intestine).

2. The pouches form when pressure inside the colon builds, usually because of constipation.

3. The main cause of diverticulosis is a low-fiber diet because it increases constipation and pressure inside the colon.

4. Most people with diverticulosis never have any discomfort or symptoms.

5. Diverticulitis occurs when the pouches get infected or inflamed and cause pain and tenderness around the left side of the lower abdomen.

6. For most people with diverticulosis, eating a high-fiber diet is the only treatment needed.

7. You can increase your fiber intake by eating these foods: whole grain breads, cereals, and other products; fruit such as

berries, apples, and peaches; and vegetables such as broccoli, cabbage, spinach, carrots, asparagus, and squash; and beans.

Chapter 20

Gallstones

Questions and Answers about Gallstones

What Are Gallstones?

Gallstones form when liquid stored in the gallbladder hardens into pieces of stone-like material. The liquid, called bile, is used to help the body digest fats. Bile is made in the liver, then stored in the gallbladder until the body needs to digest fat. At that time, the gallbladder contracts and pushes the bile into a tube—called a duct—that carries it to the small intestine, where it helps with digestion.

Bile contains water, cholesterol, fats, bile salts, and bilirubin. Bile salts break up fat, and bilirubin gives bile and stool a brownish color. If the liquid bile contains too much cholesterol, bile salts, or bilirubin, it can harden into stones.

The two types of gallstones are cholesterol stones and pigment stones. Cholesterol stones are usually yellow-green and are made primarily of hardened cholesterol. They account for about 80 percent of gallstones. Pigment stones are small, dark stones made of bilirubin. Gallstones can be as small as a grain of sand or as large as a golf ball. The gallbladder can develop just one large stone, hundreds of tiny stones, or almost any combination.

This chapter includes text from National Institute of Diabetes and Digestive and Kidney Diseases (NIDDK). NIH Publication No. 99-2897, November 1998, and "About Cholecystectomy," American College of Surgeons, 55 East Erie Street, Chicago, IL 60611; reprinted with permission.

The gallbladder and the ducts that carry bile and other digestive enzymes from the liver, gallbladder, and pancreas to the small intestine are called the **biliary system**.

Gallstones can block the normal flow of bile if they lodge in any of the ducts that carry bile from the liver to the small intestine. That includes the hepatic ducts, which carry bile out of the liver; the cystic duct, which takes bile to and from the gallbladder; and the common bile duct, which takes bile from the cystic and hepatic ducts to the small intestine. Bile trapped in these ducts can cause inflammation in the gallbladder, the ducts, or, rarely, the liver. Other ducts open into the common bile duct, including the pancreatic duct, which carries digestive enzymes out of the pancreas. If a gallstone blocks the opening to that duct, digestive enzymes can become trapped in the pancreas and cause an extremely painful inflammation called pancreatitis.

If any of these ducts remain blocked for a significant period of time, severe—possibly fatal—damage can occur, affecting the gallbladder, liver, or pancreas. Warning signs of a serious problem are fever, jaundice, and persistent pain.

What Causes Gallstones?

Cholesterol Stones. Scientists believe cholesterol stones form when bile contains too much cholesterol, too much bilirubin, or not enough bile salts, or when the gallbladder does not empty as it should for some other reason.

Pigment Stones. The cause of pigment stones is uncertain. They tend to develop in people who have cirrhosis, biliary tract infections, and hereditary blood disorders such as sickle cell anemia.

Other Factors. It is believed that the mere presence of gallstones may cause more gallstones to develop. However, other factors that contribute to gallstones have been identified, especially for cholesterol stones.

- **Obesity.** Obesity is a major risk factor for gallstones, especially in women. A large clinical study showed that being even moderately overweight increases one's risk for developing gallstones. The most likely reason is that obesity tends to reduce the amount of bile salts in bile, resulting in more cholesterol. Obesity also decreases gallbladder emptying.

- **Estrogen.** Excess estrogen from pregnancy, hormone replacement therapy, or birth control pills appears to increase cholesterol levels in bile and decrease gallbladder movement, both of which can lead to gallstones.

- **Ethnicity.** Native Americans have a genetic predisposition to secrete high levels of cholesterol in bile. In fact, they have the highest rates of gallstones in the United States. A majority of Native American men have gallstones by age 60. Among the Pima Indians of Arizona, 70 percent of women have gallstones by age 30. Mexican-American men and women of all ages also have high rates of gallstones.

- **Gender.** Women between 20 and 60 years of age are twice as likely to develop gallstones as men.

- **Age.** People over age 60 are more likely to develop gallstones than younger people.

- **Cholesterol-lowering drugs.** Drugs that lower cholesterol levels in blood actually increase the amount of cholesterol secreted in bile. This in turn can increase the risk of gallstones.

- **Diabetes.** People with diabetes generally have high levels of fatty acids called triglycerides. These fatty acids increase the risk of gallstones.

- **Rapid weight loss.** As the body metabolizes fat during rapid weight loss, it causes the liver to secrete extra cholesterol into bile, which can cause gallstones.

- **Fasting.** Fasting decreases gallbladder movement, causing the bile to become overconcentrated with cholesterol, which can lead to gallstones.

Who Is at Risk for Gallstones?

- Women.
- People over age 60.
- Native Americans.
- Mexican-Americans.
- Overweight men and women.
- People who fast or lose a lot of weight quickly.

- Pregnant women, women on hormone therapy, and women who use birth control pills.

What Are the Symptoms?

Symptoms of gallstones are often called a gallstone "attack" because they occur suddenly. A typical attack can cause:

- Steady, severe pain in the upper abdomen that increases rapidly and lasts from 30 minutes to several hours.
- Pain in the back between the shoulder blades.
- Pain under the right shoulder.
- Nausea or vomiting.

Gallstone attacks often follow fatty meals, and they may occur during the night. Other gallstone symptoms include:

- Abdominal bloating.
- Recurring intolerance of fatty foods.
- Colic.
- Belching.
- Gas.
- Indigestion.

People who also have the following symptoms should see a doctor right away:

- Sweating.
- Chills.
- Low-grade fever.
- Yellowish color of the skin or whites of the eyes.
- Clay-colored stools.

Many people with gallstones have no symptoms. These patients are said to be asymptomatic, and these stones are called "silent stones." They do not interfere in gallbladder, liver, or pancreas function and do not need treatment.

How Are Gallstones Diagnosed?

Many gallstones, especially silent stones, are discovered by accident during tests for other problems. But when gallstones are suspected to be the cause of symptoms, the doctor is likely to do an ultrasound exam. Ultrasound uses sound waves to create images of organs. Sound waves are sent toward the gallbladder through a handheld device that a technician glides over the abdomen. The sound waves bounce off the gallbladder, liver, and other organs, and their echoes make electrical impulses that create a picture of the organ on a video monitor. If stones are present, the sound waves will bounce off them, too, showing their location.

Other tests used in diagnosis include:

- **Cholecystogram or cholescintigraphy.** The patient is injected with a special iodine dye, and x-rays are taken of the gallbladder over a period of time. (Some people swallow iodine pills the night before the x-ray.) The test shows the movement of the gallbladder and any obstruction of the cystic duct.

- **Endoscopic retrograde cholangiopancreatography (ERCP).** The patient swallows an endoscope—a long, flexible, lighted tube connected to a computer and TV monitor. The doctor guides the endoscope through the stomach and into the small intestine. The doctor then injects a special dye that temporarily stains the ducts in the biliary system. ERCP is used to locate stones in the ducts.

- **Blood tests.** Blood tests may be used to look for signs of infection, obstruction, pancreatitis, or jaundice.

Gallstone symptoms are similar to those of heart attack, appendicitis, ulcers, irritable bowel syndrome, hiatal hernia, pancreatitis, and hepatitis. So accurate diagnosis is important.

What Is the Treatment?

Surgery. Surgery to remove the gallbladder is the most common way to treat symptomatic gallstones. (Asymptomatic gallstones usually do not need treatment.) Each year more than 500,000 Americans have gallbladder surgery. The surgery is called cholecystectomy.

The standard surgery is called laparoscopic cholecystectomy. For this operation, the surgeon makes several tiny incisions in the abdomen and inserts surgical instruments and a miniature video camera into the abdomen. The camera sends a magnified image from inside the body to a video monitor, giving the surgeon a closeup view of the organs and tissues. While watching the monitor, the surgeon uses the instruments to carefully separate the gallbladder from the liver, ducts, and other structures. Then the cystic duct is cut and the gallbladder removed through one of the small incisions.

Because the abdominal muscles are not cut during laparoscopic surgery, patients have less pain and fewer complications than they would have had after surgery using a large incision across the abdomen. Recovery usually involves only one night in the hospital, followed by several days of restricted activity at home.

If the surgeon discovers any obstacles to the laparoscopic procedure, such as infection or scarring from other operations, the operating team may have to switch to open surgery. In some cases the obstacles are known before surgery, and an open surgery is planned. It is called "open" surgery because the surgeon has to make a 5- to 8-inch incision in the abdomen to remove the gallbladder. This is a major surgery and may require about a 2- to 7-day stay in the hospital and several more weeks at home to recover. Open surgery is required in about 5 percent of gallbladder operations.

The most common complication in gallbladder surgery is injury to the bile ducts. An injured common bile duct can leak bile and cause a painful and potentially dangerous infection. Mild injuries can sometimes be treated nonsurgically. Major injury, however, is more serious and requires additional surgery.

If gallstones are in the bile ducts, the surgeon may use ERCP in removing them before or during the gallbladder surgery. Once the endoscope is in the small intestine, the surgeon locates the affected bile duct. An instrument on the endoscope is used to cut the duct, and the stone is captured in a tiny basket and removed with the endoscope. This two-step procedure is called ERCP with endoscopic sphincterotomy.

Occasionally, a person who has had a cholecystectomy is diagnosed with a gallstone in the bile ducts weeks, months, or even years after the surgery. The two-step ERCP procedure is usually successful in removing the stone.

Nonsurgical Treatment. Nonsurgical approaches are used only in special situations—such as when a patient's condition prevents using an anesthetic—and only for cholesterol stones. Stones recur after nonsurgical treatment about half the time.

- **Oral dissolution therapy.** Drugs made from bile acid are used to dissolve the stones. The drugs, ursodiol (Actigall) and chenodiol (Chenix), work best for small cholesterol stones. Months or years of treatment may be necessary before all the stones dissolve. Both drugs cause mild diarrhea, and chenodiol may temporarily raise levels of blood cholesterol and the liver enzyme transaminase.

- **Contact dissolution therapy.** This experimental procedure involves injecting a drug directly into the gallbladder to dissolve stones. The drug—methyl tert butyl—can dissolve some stones in 1 to 3 days, but it must be used very carefully because it is a flammable anesthetic that can be toxic. The procedure is being tested in patients with symptomatic, noncalcified cholesterol stones.

- **Extracorporeal shockwave lithotripsy (ESWL).** This treatment uses shock waves to break up stones into tiny pieces that can pass through the bile ducts without causing blockages. Attacks of biliary colic (intense pain) are common after treatment, and ESWL's success rate is not very high. Remaining stones can sometimes be dissolved with medication.

Don't People Need Their Gallbladders?

Fortunately, the gallbladder is an organ that people can live without. Losing it won't even require a change in diet. Once the gallbladder is removed, bile flows out of the liver through the hepatic ducts into the common bile duct and goes directly into the small intestine, instead of being stored in the gallbladder. However, because the bile isn't stored in the gallbladder, it flows into the small intestine more frequently, causing diarrhea in some people. Also, some studies suggest that removing the gallbladder may cause higher blood cholesterol levels, so occasional cholesterol tests may be necessary.

Points to Remember

- Gallstones form when substances in the bile harden.

- Gallstones are common among women, Native Americans, Mexican-Americans, and people who are overweight.

- Gallstone attacks often occur after eating a fatty meal.

- Symptoms can mimic those of other problems, including heart attack, so accurate diagnosis is important.

- Gallstones can cause serious problems if they become trapped in the bile ducts.

- Laparoscopic surgery to remove the gallbladder is the most common treatment.

About Cholecystectomy (Surgical Removal of the Gallbladder)

Cholecystectomy (ko-le-sis-tek'-tuh-me) is the surgical removal of the gallbladder. This section has been prepared to tell you about this operation, the conditions leading to it, and why your doctor may recommend this procedure as the best treatment for your condition.

It is important to remember that each individual is different, and the indications for the outcome of any operation depend upon the patient's individual condition. This chapter is not intended to take the place of the professional expertise of a qualified surgeon who is familiar with your symptoms. After reading this chapter, you will probably have further questions; you should discuss these openly and honestly with your surgeon.

About the Gallbladder

The gallbladder is a small, pear-shaped organ, that lies on the underside of the liver, in the right upper portion of the abdomen. It is connected by ducts (or tubes) with the liver, and with the upper portion of the small intestine (duodenum).

The liver produces bile (a substance that is essential for digesting fats) and secretes it into the gallbladder where it is concentrated and stored. When food is eaten, especially fatty or greasy foods, the gallbladder contracts and forces bile out the ducts leading into the intestine. When the gallbladder is removed, this function is taken over by the liver and its ducts.

Gallbladder Disease

Frequently, the gallbladder contains stones or develops an infection that can interfere with its role in the digestive process. The exact causes of these conditions are not known.

Anyone can develop gallbladder disease, but it is more common in people who are overweight, and between the ages of 35 and 55. Women are more likely to suffer from it than men, a factor which appears to be associated with metabolic changes that take place during pregnancy.

Symptoms of Gallbladder Disease

Sometimes, persons with gallbladder disease have few or no symptoms. Some, however, will eventually develop one or more of the following symptoms:

1. Frequent bouts of indigestion, especially after eating fatty or greasy foods, or certain vegetables such as cabbage, radishes, or pickles.

2. Nausea, heartburn, and bloating.

3. Attacks of sharp pains in the upper right part of the abdomen. This pain occurs when a gallstone becomes lodged in the duct from the gallbladder to the intestine.

4. Jaundice (yellowing of the skin) may occur if a gallstone becomes stuck in the common bile duct which leads into the intestine, blocking the entire flow of bile from both the gallbladder and the liver. This is a serious complication and usually requires an immediate emergency operation.

Diagnosing Gallbladder Disease

Because the majority of patients who have gallbladder disease also have gallstones, the diagnosis can usually be confirmed through the use of ultrasound, a safe and painless technique that uses high frequency sound waves to project an image of the gallbladder and gallstones on a special screen.

There are some occasions, however, when ultrasound cannot confirm a diagnosis in patients who have symptomatic gallbladder disease. Therefore, other diagnostic methods may be used, such as through the use of x-rays or various other types of scanning methods.

Treating Gallbladder Disease

The only curative treatment for gallbladder disease is surgical removal of the gallbladder. Generally, when stones are present and causing symptoms, or when the gallbladder is infected and inflamed, removal of the organ is usually necessary.

When the gallbladder is removed, the surgeon also examines the bile ducts, sometimes with x-rays, and removes any stones that may be lodged there. The ducts are not removed so that the liver can continue to secrete bile into the intestine, taking over the function of the gallbladder.

Most patients experience no further symptoms after cholecystectomy. However, mild residual symptoms are not uncommon. They can usually be controlled with a special diet and medication.

There are two commonly performed procedures for removal of the gallbladder. These are called laparoscopic (lap"ah-ro-skop'ic) cholecystectomy and conventional cholecystectomy. Discuss with your surgeon which operation is best for your condition.

About Laparoscopic Cholecystectomy

In this procedure, the surgeon uses video technology and highly specialized tools to remove the gallbladder without making a large surgical incision.

Instead, the surgeon creates four very small incisions of less than half an inch each. One of these holes is made in or near the patient's navel so that the surgeon can insert a special instrument called the laparoscope (lap'ah-ro-skop"). The laparoscope is a long, rigid tube that is attached to a tiny video camera and a light. Before the laparoscope is inserted, the patient's abdomen is distended with an injection of carbon dioxide gas which allows the surgeon to see inside the body. Once the laparoscope has been inserted, the surgeon then guides the laparoscope while watching the view it provides on two video monitors.

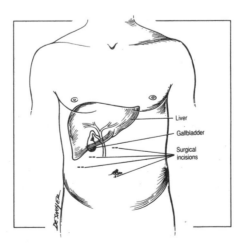

Figure 20.1. *During laparoscopic cholecystectomy the surgeon makes four very small incisions of less than half an inch each.*

The other incisions are made in the abdomen, two of them are on the right side below the ribcage, and one is in the upper portion at the midline. Each of these three incisions is used for other specialized instruments. Two are used to grasp and retract the gallbladder and the third to insert instruments to free the gallbladder from its attachments.

The instrument that cuts the gallbladder free may be either a surgical laser or an electrocautery device. Both procedures employ localized heat to prevent bleeding. Whichever tools your surgeon elects to use, you can feel comfortable in knowing that the procedure has been proven safe and effective in thousands of similar operations.

Once the gallbladder has been cut free, the surgeon drains it of bile, collapses the organ, and removes it through the incision at the navel. After the operation, patients are often back on their feet and on their way home the very next day. Many return to work within a week. Once healed, the scars left from the four incisions are so small that they are barely noticeable.

In about one in 20 cases during a laparoscopic operation, the surgeon discovers a problem, such as a severely diseased gallbladder or an excessive amount of inflammation, that requires the performance of a conventional operation (see below). Because the surgeon cannot see the gallbladder in detail until the laparoscope is inserted during the operation, some complications cannot be predicted and are only discovered once the operation has begun. Thus, patients should always be prepared for the possibility of having to undergo a conventional cholecystectomy.

About Conventional Cholecystectomy

In conventional cholecystectomy, the surgeon makes an incision that is approximately four to six inches long. The incision is made either longitudinally (up and down) in the upper portion of the abdomen, or obliquely (at a slant) beneath the ribs on the right side.

During the operation, drains may be inserted into the wound, which will be removed while the patient is still in the hospital.

During the operation, the surgeon may also remove the appendix. This is a preventive measure to avoid a possible future operation for appendicitis.

In uncomplicated situations, the hospital stay following conventional gallbladder surgery is about four to seven days. Most patients can get out of bed the day of the operation, and can return to normal activity within four weeks or less. In more complicated cases, patients may resume normal activity within four to eight weeks.

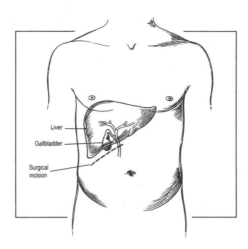

Figure 20.2. *During conventional cholecystectomy the surgeon makes an incision that is approximately four to six inches long.*

Removal of the gallbladder is one of the most common surgical procedures. Whichever procedure your surgeon recommends (a conventional operation or a laparoscopic cholecystectomy), you can be confident in knowing that these are not considered dangerous or risky operations in otherwise healthy individuals.

—Reviewed By: Charles K. McSherry, MD, FACS,
Director of Surgery, Beth Israel Medical Center, New York, NY

Surgery by Surgeons

A fully trained surgeon is a physician who, after medical school, has gone through years of training in an accredited residency program to learn the specialized skills of a surgeon. One good sign of a surgeon's competence is certification by a national surgical board approved by the American Board of Medical Specialties. All board-certified surgeons have satisfactorily completed an approved residency training program and have passed a rigorous specialty examination.

The letters F.A.C.S. (Fellow of the American College of Surgeons) after a surgeon's name are a further indication of a physician's qualifications. Surgeons who become Fellows of the College have passed a comprehensive evaluation of their surgical training and skills; they also have demonstrated their commitment to high standards of ethical conduct. This evaluation is conducted according to national standards that were established to ensure that patients receive the best possible surgical care.

Prepared as a public service by the American College of Surgeons.

American College of Surgeons
55 East Erie Street
Chicago, IL 60611

Chapter 21

Gas in the Digestive Tract

Why Do I Have Gas?

Everyone has gas and eliminates it by burping or passing it through the rectum. However, many people think they have too much gas when they really have normal amounts. Most people produce about 1 to 3 pints a day and pass gas about 14 times a day.

Gas is made primarily of odorless vapors—carbon dioxide, oxygen, nitrogen, hydrogen, and sometimes methane. The unpleasant odor of flatulence comes from bacteria in the large intestine that release small amounts of gases that contain sulfur.

Although having gas is common, it can be uncomfortable and embarrassing. Understanding causes, ways to reduce symptoms, and treatment will help most people find relief.

What Causes Gas?

Gas in the digestive tract (that is, the esophagus, stomach, small intestine, and large intestine) comes from two sources:

- Swallowed air

- Normal breakdown of certain undigested foods by harmless bacteria naturally present in the large intestine (colon).

National Institute of Diabetes and Digestive and Kidney Diseases (NIDDK), NIH Pub. No. 97-883, updated November 1998.

159

Swallowed Air

Air swallowing (aerophagia) is a common cause of gas in the stomach. Everyone swallows small amounts of air when eating and drinking. However, eating or drinking rapidly, chewing gum, smoking, or wearing loose dentures can cause some people to take in more air.

Burping, or belching, is the way most swallowed air—which contains nitrogen, oxygen, and carbon dioxide—leaves the stomach. The remaining gas moves into the small intestine where it is partially absorbed. A small amount travels into the large intestine for release through the rectum. (The stomach also releases carbon dioxide when stomach acid and bicarbonate mix, but most of this gas is absorbed into the bloodstream and does not enter the large intestine.)

Breakdown of Undigested Foods

The body does not digest and absorb some carbohydrates (the sugar, starches, and fiber found in many foods) in the small intestine because of a shortage or absence of certain enzymes.

This undigested food then passes from the small intestine into the large intestine, where harmless and normal bacteria break down the food, producing hydrogen, carbon dioxide, and, in about one-third of all people, methane. Eventually these gases exit through the rectum.

People who make methane do not necessarily pass more gas or have unique symptoms. A person who produces methane will have stools that consistently float in water. Research has not shown why some people produce methane and others do not.

Foods that produce gas in one person may not cause gas in another. Some common bacteria in the large intestine can destroy the hydrogen that other bacteria produce. The balance of the two types of bacteria may explain why some people have more gas than others.

Which Foods Cause Gas?

Most foods that contain carbohydrates can cause gas. By contrast, fats and proteins cause little gas.

Sugars

The sugars that cause gas are: raffinose, lactose, fructose, and sorbitol.

Raffinose. Beans contain large amounts of this complex sugar. Smaller amounts are found in cabbage, Brussels sprouts, broccoli, asparagus, other vegetables, and whole grains.

Lactose. Lactose is the natural sugar in milk. It is also found in milk products, such as cheese and ice cream, and processed foods, such as bread, cereal, and salad dressing. Many people, particularly those of African, Native American, or Asian background, have low levels of the enzyme lactase needed to digest lactose. Also, as people age, their enzyme levels decrease. As a result, over time people may experience increasing amounts of gas after eating food containing lactose.

Fructose. Fructose is naturally present in onions, artichokes, pears, and wheat. It is also used as a sweetener in some soft drinks and fruit drinks.

Sorbitol. Sorbitol is a sugar found naturally in fruits, including apples, pears, peaches, and prunes. It is also used as an artificial sweetener in many dietetic foods and sugar free candies and gums.

Starches

Most starches, including potatoes, corn, noodles, and wheat, produce gas as they are broken down in the large intestine. Rice is the only starch that does not cause gas.

Fiber

Many foods contain soluble and insoluble fiber. Soluble fiber dissolves easily in water and takes on a soft, gel-like texture in the intestines. Found in oat bran, beans, peas, and most fruits, soluble fiber is not broken down until it reaches the large intestine where digestion causes gas.

Insoluble fiber, on the other hand, passes essentially unchanged through the intestines and produces little gas. Wheat bran and some vegetables contain this kind of fiber.

What Are Some Symptoms and Problems of Gas?

The most common symptoms of gas are belching, flatulence, abdominal bloating, and abdominal pain. However, not everyone experiences these symptoms. The determining factors probably are how much gas the body produces, how many fatty acids the body absorbs, and a person's sensitivity to gas in the large intestine. Chronic symptoms caused by too much gas or by a serious disease are rare.

Belching

An occasional belch during or after meals is normal and releases gas when the stomach is full of food. However, people who belch frequently may be swallowing too much air and releasing it before the air enters the stomach.

Sometimes a person with chronic belching may have an upper GI disorder, such as peptic ulcer disease, gastroesophageal reflux disease (GERD), or gastritis.

Believing that swallowing air and releasing it will relieve the discomfort of these disorders, this person may unintentionally develop a habitual cycle of belching and discomfort. Frequently, the pain continues or worsens, leading the person to believe he or she has a serious disorder.

Two rare chronic gas syndromes are associated with belching: Meganblase syndrome and gas-bloat syndrome. The Meganblase syndrome, which causes chronic belching, is characterized by severe air swallowing and an enlarged bubble of gas in the stomach following heavy meals. The resulting fullness and shortness of breath may mimic a heart attack.

Gas-bloat syndrome may occur after surgery to correct GERD. The surgery creates a one-way valve between the esophagus and stomach that allows food and gas to enter the stomach but often prevents normal belching and the ability to vomit.

Flatulence

Another common complaint is passage of too much gas through the rectum (flatulence). However, most people do not realize that passing gas 14 to 23 times a day is normal. Although rare, too much gas may be the result of severe carbohydrate malabsorption or overactive bacteria in the colon.

Abdominal Bloating

Many people believe that too much gas causes abdominal bloating. However, people who complain of bloating from gas often have normal amounts and distribution of gas. They actually may be unusually aware of gas in the digestive tract.

Doctors believe that bloating is usually the result of an intestinal motility disorder, such as IBS. Motility disorders are characterized by abnormal movements and contractions of intestinal muscles. These disorders may give a false sensation of bloating because of increased sensitivity to gas.

Splenic-flexure syndrome is a chronic disorder that seems to be caused by trapped gas at bends (flexures) in the colon. Symptoms include bloating, muscle spasms, and upper abdominal discomfort. Splenic-flexure syndrome often accompanies IBS.

Any disease that causes intestinal obstruction, such as Crohn's disease or colon cancer, may also cause abdominal bloating. In addition, people who have had many operations, adhesions (scar tissue), or internal hernias may experience bloating or pain. Finally, eating a lot of fatty food can delay stomach emptying and cause bloating and discomfort, but not necessarily too much gas.

Abdominal Pain and Discomfort

Some people have pain when gas is present in the intestine. When gas collects on the left side of the colon, the pain can be confused with heart disease. When it collects on the right side of the colon, the pain may feel like the pain associated with gallstones or appendicitis.

What Diagnostic Tests Are Used?

Because gas symptoms may be caused by a serious disorder, those causes should be ruled out. The doctor usually begins with a review of dietary habits and symptoms. The doctor may ask the patient to keep a diary of foods and beverages consumed for a specific time period.

If lactase deficiency is the suspected cause of gas, the doctor may suggest avoiding milk products for a period of time. A blood or breath test may be used to diagnose lactose intolerance.

In addition, to determine if someone produces too much gas in the colon or is unusually sensitive to the passage of normal gas volumes, the doctor may ask patients to count the number of times they pass gas during the day and include this information in a diary.

Careful review of diet and the amount of gas passed may help relate specific foods to symptoms and determine the severity of the problem.

If a patient complains of bloating, the doctor may examine the abdomen for the sound of fluid movement to rule out ascites (build up of fluid in the abdomen) and for signs of inflammation to rule out diseases of the colon.

The possibility of colon cancer is usually considered in people 50 years of age and older and in those with a family history of colorectal cancer, particularly if they have never had a colon examination (sigmoidoscopy or colonoscopy). These tests may also be appropriate for someone with unexplained weight loss, diarrhea, or blood not visible in the stool.

For those with chronic belching, the doctor will look for signs or causes of excessive air swallowing. If needed, an upper GI series (x-ray to view the esophagus, stomach, and upper small intestine) may be performed to rule out disease.

How Is Gas Treated?

The most common ways to reduce the discomfort of gas are changing diet, taking medicines, and reducing the amount of air swallowed.

Diet

Doctors may tell people to eat fewer foods that cause gas. However, for some people this may mean cutting out healthy foods, such as fruits and vegetables, whole grains, and milk products.

Doctors may also suggest limiting high-fat foods to reduce bloating and discomfort. This helps the stomach empty faster, allowing gases to move into the small intestine.

Unfortunately, the amount of gas caused by certain foods varies from person to person. Effective dietary changes depend on learning through trial and error how much of the offending foods one can handle.

Nonprescription Medicines

Many nonprescription, over-the-counter medicines are available to help reduce symptoms, including antacids with simethicone and activated charcoal. Digestive enzymes, such as lactase supplements, actually help digest carbohydrates and may allow people to eat foods that normally cause gas.

Antacids, such as Mylanta II, Maalox II and Di-Gel, contain simethicone, a foaming agent that joins gas bubbles in the stomach so that gas is more easily belched away. However, these medicines have no effect on intestinal gas. The recommended dose is 2 to 4 tablespoons of the simethicone preparation taken 1/2 to 2 hours after meals.

Activated charcoal tablets (Charcocaps) may provide relief from gas in the colon. Studies have shown that when taken before and after a meal, intestinal gas is greatly reduced. The usual dose is 2 to 4 tablets taken just before eating and 1 hour after meals.

The enzyme lactase, which aids with lactose digestion, is available in liquid and tablet form without a prescription (Lactaid, Lactrase, and Dairy Ease). Adding a few drops of liquid lactase to milk before drinking it or chewing lactase tablets just before eating helps digest foods that contain lactose. Also, lactose-reduced milk and other products are available at many grocery stores (Lactaid and Dairy Ease).

Beano, a newer over-the-counter digestive aid, contains the sugar-digesting enzyme that the body lacks to digest the sugar in beans and many vegetables. The enzyme comes in liquid form. Three to 10 drops are added per serving just before eating to break down the gas-producing sugars. Beano has no effect on gas caused by lactose or fiber.

Prescription Medicines

Doctors may prescribe medicines to help reduce symptoms, especially for people with a motility disorder, such as IBS. Promotility or prokinetic drugs, such as metoclopramide (Reglan) and cisapride (Propulsid), may move gas through the digestive tract quickly.

Reducing Swallowed Air

For those who have chronic belching, doctors may suggest ways to reduce the amount of air swallowed. Recommendations are to avoid chewing gum and to avoid eating hard candy. Eating at a slow pace and checking with a dentist to make sure dentures fit properly should also help.

Conclusion

Although gas may be uncomfortable and embarrassing, it is not life-threatening. Understanding causes, ways to reduce symptoms, and treatment will help most people find some relief.

Points to Remember

1. Everyone has gas in the digestive tract.

2. People often believe normal passage of gas to be excessive.

3. Gas comes from two main sources: swallowed air and normal breakdown of certain foods by harmless bacteria naturally present in the large intestine.

4. Many foods with carbohydrates can cause gas. Fats and proteins cause little gas.

5. Foods that may cause gas include:

   - Beans

   - Vegetables, such as broccoli, cabbage, Brussels sprouts, onions, artichokes, and asparagus

   - Fruits, such as pears, apples, and peaches

   - Whole grains, such as whole wheat and bran

   - Soft drinks and fruit drinks

   - Milk and milk products, such as cheese and ice cream, and packaged foods prepared with lactose, such as bread, cereal, and salad dressing

   - Foods containing sorbitol, such as dietetic foods and sugar-free candies and gums.

6. The most common symptoms of gas are belching, flatulence, bloating, and abdominal pain. However, some of these symptoms are often caused by an intestinal motility disorder, such as irritable bowel syndrome, rather than too much gas.

7. The most common ways to reduce the discomfort of gas are changing diet, taking nonprescription or prescription medicines, and reducing the amount of air swallowed.

8. Digestive enzymes, such as lactase supplements, actually help digest carbohydrates and may allow people to eat foods that normally cause gas.

Chapter 22

Heartburn (Gastroesophageal Reflux Disease)

Introduction

Gastroesophageal reflux disease (GERD) is a digestive disorder that affects the lower esophageal sphincter (LES)—the muscle connecting the esophagus with the stomach. Many people, including pregnant women, suffer from heartburn or acid indigestion caused by GERD. Doctors believe that some people suffer from GERD due to a condition called hiatal hernia. In most cases, heartburn can be relieved through diet and lifestyle changes; however, some people may require medication or surgery. This chapter provides information on GERD—its causes, symptoms, treatment, and long-term complications.

Questions and Answers about GERD

What Is Gastroesophageal Reflux?

Gastroesophageal refers to the stomach and esophagus. Reflux means to flow back or return. Therefore, gastroesophageal reflux is the return of the stomach's contents back up into the esophagus.

In normal digestion, the LES opens to allow food to pass into the stomach and closes to prevent food and acidic stomach juices from flowing back into the esophagus. Gastroesophageal reflux occurs when

National Institute of Diabetes and Digestive and Kidney Diseases (NIDDK). NIH Publication No. 94-882, September 1994.

the LES is weak or relaxes inappropriately allowing the stomach's contents to flow up into the esophagus. Figure 22.1 shows the location of the LES between the esophagus and the stomach.

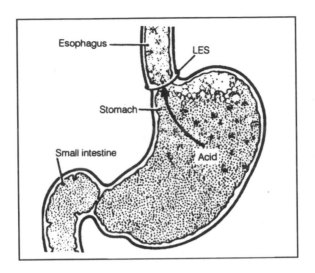

Figure 22.1.

The severity of GERD depends on LES dysfunction as well as the type and amount of fluid brought up from the stomach and the neutralizing effect of saliva.

What Is the Role of Hiatal Hernia?

Some doctors believe a hiatal hernia may weaken the LES and cause reflux. Hiatal hernia occurs when the upper part of the stomach moves up into the chest through a small opening in the diaphragm (diaphragmatic hiatus). The diaphragm is the muscle separating the stomach from the chest. (See Figure 22.2.) Recent studies show that the opening in the diaphragm acts as an additional sphincter around the lower end of the esophagus. Studies also show that hiatal hernia results in retention of acid and other contents above this opening. These substances can reflux easily into the esophagus.

Coughing, vomiting, straining, or sudden physical exertion can cause increased pressure in the abdomen resulting in hiatal hernia.

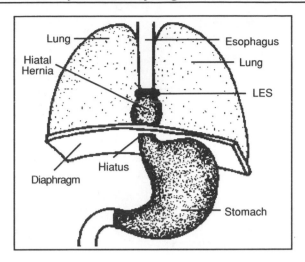

Figure 22.2.

Obesity and pregnancy also contribute to this condition. Many otherwise healthy people age 50 and over have a small hiatal hernia. Although considered a condition of middle age, hiatal hernias affect people of all ages.

Hiatal hernias usually do not require treatment. However, treatment may be necessary if the hernia is in danger of becoming strangulated (twisted in a way that cuts off blood supply, i.e., paraesophageal hernia) or is complicated by severe GERD or esophagitis(inflammation of the esophagus). The doctor may perform surgery to reduce the size of the hernia or to prevent strangulation.

What Other Factors Contribute to GERD?

Dietary and lifestyle choices may contribute to GERD. Certain foods and beverages, including chocolate, peppermint, fried or fatty foods, coffee, or alcoholic beverages, may weaken the LES causing reflux and heartburn. Studies show that cigarette smoking relaxes the LES. Obesity and pregnancy can also cause GERD.

What Does Heartburn Feel Like?

Heartburn, also called acid indigestion, is the most common symptom of GERD and usually feels like a burning chest pain beginning behind the breastbone and moving upward to the neck and throat. Many people say it feels like food is coming back into the mouth leaving an acid or bitter taste.

The burning, pressure, or pain of heartburn can last as long as 2 hours and is often worse after eating. Lying down or bending over can also result in heartburn. Many people obtain relief by standing upright or by taking an antacid that clears acid out of the esophagus.

Heartburn pain can be mistaken for the pain associated with heart disease or a heart attack, but there are differences. Exercise may aggravate pain resulting from heart disease, and rest may relieve the pain. Heartburn pain is less likely to be associated with physical activity.

How Common Is Heartburn?

More than 60 million American adults experience GERD and heartburn at least once a month, and about 25 million adults suffer daily from heartburn. Twenty-five percent of pregnant women experience daily heartburn, and more than 50 percent have occasional distress. Recent studies show that GERD in infants and children is more common than previously recognized and may produce recurrent vomiting, coughing and other respiratory problems, or failure to thrive.

What Is the Treatment for GERD?

Doctors recommend lifestyle and dietary changes for most people with GERD. Treatment aims at decreasing the amount of reflux or reducing damage to the lining of the esophagus from refluxed materials.

Avoiding foods and beverages that can weaken the LES is recommended. These foods include chocolate, peppermint, fatty foods, coffee, and alcoholic beverages. Foods and beverages that can irritate a damaged esophageal lining, such as citrus fruits and juices, tomato products, and pepper, should also be avoided.

Decreasing the size of portions at mealtime may also help control symptoms. Eating meals at least 2 to 3 hours before bedtime may lessen reflux by allowing the acid in the stomach to decrease and the stomach to empty partially. In addition, being overweight often worsens symptoms. Many overweight people find relief when they lose weight.

Cigarette smoking weakens the LES. Therefore, stopping smoking is important to reduce GERD symptoms.

Elevating the head of the bed on 6-inch blocks or sleeping on a specially designed wedge reduces heartburn by allowing gravity to minimize reflux of stomach contents into the esophagus.

Antacids taken regularly can neutralize acid in the esophagus and stomach and stop heartburn. Many people find that nonprescription antacids provide temporary or partial relief. An antacid combined with a foaming agent such as alginic acid helps some people. These compounds are believed to form a foam barrier on top of the stomach that prevents acid reflux from occurring.

Long-term use of antacids, however, can result in side effects, including diarrhea, altered calcium metabolism (a change in the way the body breaks down and uses calcium), and buildup of magnesium in the body. Too much magnesium can be serious for patients with kidney disease. If antacids are needed for more than 3 weeks, a doctor should be consulted.

For chronic reflux and heartburn, the doctor may prescribe medications to reduce acid in the stomach. These medicines include H2 blockers, which inhibit acid secretion in the stomach. Currently, four H2 blockers are available: cimetidine, famotidine, nizatidine, and ranitidine. Another type of drug, the proton pump (or acid pump) inhibitor omeprazole inhibits an enzyme (a protein in the acid-producing cells of the stomach) necessary for acid secretion. The acid pump inhibitor lansoprazole is currently under investigation as a new treatment for GERD.

Other approaches to therapy will increase the strength of the LES and quicken emptying of stomach contents with motility drugs that act on the upper gastrointestinal (GI) tract. These drugs include cisapride, bethanechol, and metoclopramide.

Tips to Control Heartburn

1. Avoid foods and beverages that affect LES pressure or irritate the esophagus lining, including fried and fatty foods, peppermint, chocolate, alcohol, coffee, citrus fruit and juices, and tomato products.

2. Lose weight if overweight.

3. Stop smoking.

4. Elevate the head of the bed 6 inches.

5. Avoid lying down 2 to 3 hours after eating.

6. Take an antacid.

What If Symptoms Persist?

People with severe, chronic esophageal reflux or with symptoms not relieved by the treatment described above may need more complete diagnostic evaluation. Doctors use a variety of tests and procedures to examine a patient with chronic heartburn.

An *upper GI series* may be performed during the early phase of testing. This test is a special x-ray that shows the esophagus, stomach, and duodenum (the upper part of the small intestine). While an upper GI series provides limited information about possible reflux, it is used to rule out other diagnoses, such as peptic ulcers.

Endoscopy is an important procedure for individuals with chronic GERD. By placing a small lighted tube with a tiny video camera on the end (endoscope) into the esophagus, the doctor may see inflammation or irritation of the tissue lining the esophagus (esophagitis). If the findings of the endoscopy are abnormal or questionable, biopsy (removing a small sample of tissue) from the lining of the esophagus may be helpful.

The *Bernstein test* (dripping a mild acid through a tube placed in the mid-esophagus) is often performed as part of a complete evaluation. This test attempts to confirm that the symptoms result from acid in the esophagus.

Esophageal manometric studies—pressure measurements of the esophagus—occasionally help identify critically low pressure in the LES or abnormalities in esophageal muscle contraction.

For patients in whom diagnosis is difficult, doctors may measure the acid levels inside the esophagus through pH testing. Testing pH monitors the acidity level of the esophagus and symptoms during meals, activity, and sleep. Newer techniques of long-term pH monitoring are improving diagnostic capability in this area.

Does GERD Require Surgery?

A small number of people with GERD may need surgery because of severe reflux and poor response to medical treatment. Fundoplication is a surgical procedure that increases pressure in the lower esophagus. However, surgery should not be considered until all other measures have been tried.

What Are the Complications of Long-Term GERD?

Sometimes GERD results in serious complications. Esophagitis can occur as a result of too much stomach acid in the esophagus.

Esophagitis may cause esophageal bleeding or ulcers. In addition, a narrowing or stricture of the esophagus may occur from chronic scarring. Some people develop a condition known as Barrett's esophagus, which is severe damage to the skin-like lining of the esophagus. Doctors believe this condition may be a precursor to esophageal cancer.

Conclusion

Although GERD can limit daily activities and productivity, it is rarely life-threatening. With an understanding of the causes and proper treatment most people will find relief.

Additional Readings

Cramer T. A burning question: When do you need an antacid? *FDA Consumer* 1992; 26(1): 19-22. This article for consumers provides general information about antacids.

Larson DE, Editor-in-chief. *Mayo Clinic Family Health Book*. New York: William Morrow and Company, Inc., 1990. This general medical guide includes sections about esophageal reflux and hiatal hernia.

Richter JE. Why does surgery work for GERD? *Practical Gastroenterology* 1993; XVII(10): 10-18. This article for physicians describes antireflux surgery.

Sutherland JE. Gastroesophageal reflux disease: when antacids aren't enough. *Postgraduate Medicine* 1991; 89(7): 45-53. This article for primary care physicians provides guidelines to determine if a patient has reflux disease and offers treatment methods.

Chapter 23

Hemorrhoids

What Are Hemorrhoids?

Hemorrhoids are swollen but normally present blood vessels in and around the anus and lower rectum that stretch under pressure, similar to varicose veins in the legs.

The increased pressure and swelling may result from straining to move the bowel. Other contributing factors include pregnancy, heredity, aging, and chronic constipation or diarrhea.

Hemorrhoids are either inside the anus (internal) or under the skin around the anus (external).

What Are the Symptoms of Hemorrhoids?

Many anorectal problems, including fissures, fistulae, abscesses, or irritation and itching (pruritus ani), have similar symptoms and are incorrectly referred to as hemorrhoids.

Hemorrhoids usually are not dangerous or life threatening. In most cases, hemorrhoidal symptoms will go away within a few days.

Although many people have hemorrhoids, not all experience symptoms. The most common symptom of internal hemorrhoids is bright red blood covering the stool, on toilet paper, or in the toilet bowl. However, an internal hemorrhoid may protrude through the anus outside the body, becoming irritated and painful. This is known as a protruding hemorrhoid.

National Institutes of Diabetes and Digestive and Kidney Disorders (NIDDK), NIH Pub No. 95-3201, updated November 1998.

Symptoms of external hemorrhoids may include painful swelling or a hard lump around the anus that results when a blood clot forms. This condition is known as a thrombosed external hemorrhoid.

In addition, excessive straining, rubbing, or cleaning around the anus may cause irritation with bleeding and/or itching, which may produce a vicious cycle of symptoms. Draining mucus may also cause itching.

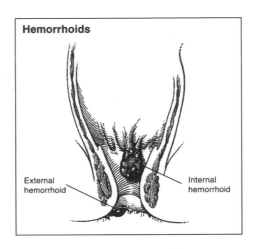

Figure 23.1. *Two Types of Hemorrhoid: Internal and External*

How Common Are Hemorrhoids?

Hemorrhoids are very common in men and women. About half of the population have hemorrhoids by age 50. Hemorrhoids are also common among pregnant women. The pressure of the fetus in the abdomen, as well as hormonal changes, cause the hemorrhoidal vessels to enlarge. These vessels are also placed under severe pressure during childbirth. For most women, however, hemorrhoids caused by pregnancy are a temporary problem.

How Are Hemorrhoids Diagnosed?

A thorough evaluation and proper diagnosis by the doctor is important any time bleeding from the rectum or blood in the stool lasts more than a couple of days. Bleeding may also be a symptom of other digestive diseases, including colorectal cancer.

The doctor will examine the anus and rectum to look for swollen blood vessels that indicate hemorrhoids and will also perform a digital rectal exam with a gloved, lubricated finger to feel for abnormalities.

Closer evaluation of the rectum for hemorrhoids requires an exam with an anoscope, a hollow, lighted tube useful for viewing internal hemorrhoids, or a proctoscope, useful for more completely examining the entire rectum.

To rule out other causes of gastrointestinal bleeding, the doctor may examine the rectum and lower colon (sigmoid) with sigmoidoscopy or the entire colon with colonoscopy. Sigmoidoscopy and colonoscopy are diagnostic procedures that also involve the use of lighted, flexible tubes inserted through the rectum.

What Is the Treatment?

Medical treatment of hemorrhoids initially is aimed at relieving symptoms. Measures to reduce symptoms include:

- Warm tub or sitz baths several times a day in plain, warm water for about 10 minutes.

- Ice packs to help reduce swelling.

- Application of a hemorroidal cream or suppository to the affected area for a limited time.

Prevention of the recurrence of hemorrhoids is aimed at changing conditions associated with the pressure and straining of constipation. Doctors will often recommend increasing fiber and fluids in the diet. Eating the right amount of fiber and drinking six to eight glasses of fluid (not alcohol) result in softer, bulkier stools. A softer stool makes emptying the bowels easier and lessens the pressure on hemorrhoids caused by straining. Eliminating straining also helps prevent the hemorrhoids from protruding.

Good sources of fiber are fruits, vegetables, and whole grains. In addition, doctors may suggest a bulk stool softener or a fiber supplement such aspsyllium (Metamucil) or methylcellulose (Citrucel).

In some cases, hemorrhoids must be treated surgically. These methods are used to shrink and destroy the hemorrhoidal tissue and are performed under anesthesia. The doctor will perform the surgery during an office or hospital visit.

A number of surgical methods may be used to remove or reduce the size of internal hemorrhoids. These techniques include:

- Rubber band ligation—A rubber band is placed around the base of the hemorrhoid inside the rectum. The band cuts off circulation, and the hemorrhoid withers away within a few days.

- Sclerotherapy—A chemical solution is injected around the blood vessel to shrink the hemorrhoid.

Techniques used to treat both internal and external hemorrhoids include:

- Electrical or laser heat (laser coagulation) or infrared light (infrared photo coagulation)—Both techniques use special devices to burn hemorrhoidal tissue.

- Hemorrhoidectomy—Occasionally, extensive or severe internal or external hemorrhoids may require removal by surgery known as hemorrhoidectomy. This is the best method for permanent removal of hemorrhoids.

How Are Hemorrhoids Prevented?

The best way to prevent hemorrhoids is to keep stools soft so they pass easily, thus decreasing pressure and straining, and to empty bowels as soon as possible after the urge occurs. Exercise, including walking, and increased fiber in the diet help reduce constipation and straining by producing stools that are softer and easier to pass. In addition, a person should not sit on the toilet for a long period of time.

Chapter 24

Hernias

A hernia (her'-ne-ah) occurs when a small sac containing tissue protrudes through an opening in the muscles of the abdominal wall. The technical name for the operation that repairs a hernia is called a herniorrhaphy (her" ne-or'ah-fe). This chapter will explain:

- Why you may need to have a hernia repaired
- The ways in which a hernia can be corrected surgically
- What to expect before and after the operation

Remember, as routine as a hernia repair is (over half a million operations were done in the US last year [1993]), no two people undergoing a herniorrhaphy are alike. The reasons for and the outcome of any operation depend on your overall health, your age, the severity and size of your hernia, and the strength of your abdominal tissues.

This chapter is not intended to take the place of your doctor's professional opinion. Rather, it can help you begin to understand the basics of these surgical procedures. Read this material carefully. If you have additional questions, you should discuss them openly with your doctor.

About Hernias

A hernia develops when the outer layers of the abdominal wall weaken, bulge, or actually rip. The hole in this outer layer allows the

179

inner lining of the cavity to protrude and to form a sac. Any part of the abdominal wall can develop a hernia. However, the most common site is the groin. A hernia in the groin area is called an inguinal (ing'gwi-nal) hernia (inguinal is another word for groin). Inguinal hernias account for 80 percent of all hernias. In an inguinal hernia, the sac protrudes into the groin toward—and sometimes into—the scrotum. Although most common in men, groin hernias can also occur in women.

Another type of hernia develops through the navel, and it is called an umbilical hernia. A hernia that pushes through past a surgical incision or operation site is called an incisional hernia. A hiatal hernia forms when the upper portion of the stomach slides into the chest cavity through the normal opening created by the esophagus, or food pipe.

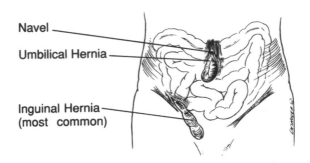

Figure 24.1. Common hernia locations.

Who Gets Hernias?

Most inguinal hernias in adults result from strain on the abdominal muscles, which have been weakened by age or by congenital factors. The types of activity associated with the appearance of an inguinal hernia include:

- Lifting heavy objects
- Sudden twists, pulls, or muscle strains
- Marked gains in weight, causing an increase in pressure on the abdominal wall
- Chronic constipation, which places a strain on the abdomen while on the toilet

- Repeated attacks of coughing

A hernia is called reducible if the protruding sac of tissue can be pushed back into place inside the abdomen. If the hernia cannot be pushed back, it is called irreducible, incarcerated, or imprisoned.

The symptoms of inguinal hernias vary. Sometimes the onset is gradual, with no symptoms other than the development of a bulge. Other times, the hernia will occur suddenly with a feeling that something has "given way." This feeling can be accompanied by pain or discomfort. Signs and symptoms of inguinal hernias can include:

- Visible bulges in the scrotum, groin, or abdominal wall
- A feeling of weakness or pressure in the groin
- A burning feeling at the bulge
- A gurgling feeling

In some cases, an irreducible hernia gets so pinched that the blood supply is cut off and the tissue swells. Rapidly worsening pain or a tender lump is a signal that the hernia has strangulated. When strangulation occurs, the tissue can die quickly and become infected. Within hours this condition can lead to a life-threatening medical emergency that requires immediate medical attention.

Preparing for the Operation

Unless the hernia is strangulated, hernia repair typically is an elective operation. Only you can decide whether you ought to proceed with the repair. However, you must realize that (1) the hernia is not going to heal by itself and (2) pain may increase in the area of the hernia, and it will usually increase in size over time.

Prior to admission to the hospital, you may be given standard tests to measure your complete blood count and electrolyte levels, as well as a urinalysis. Your surgeon may require additional studies depending on your condition and age. Prior to the operation, you will dress in a surgical cap and gown, receive a sedative by injection, and have a needle placed in the back of your hand or in your forearm for connection to an intravenous line in the operating room. In addition, the area where your incision will be made will be shaved. The procedure generally takes less than two hours. You may be given a local, spinal, or general anesthetic depending on your surgeon's preference, your age, your state of health, and the procedure's degree of difficulty.

Outpatient Surgery

Unless there is cause for concern, hernia repair can be done on an outpatient basis. On the day of your operation, you should wear loose-fitting, simple clothing to the hospital, such as a sweat suit and slip-on shoes. That way, upon discharge, you will be able to get dressed easily without too much strain or discomfort. Generally, you should not eat on the morning of your operation. You should have a friend or relative drive you home after the operation and, ideally, someone should stay with you the first night, particularly if your bedroom is on the second floor of your house because stairs will be difficult for you to climb.

Types of Procedures

Today, surgeons are performing a variety of techniques to repair hernias. You should talk with your surgeon to determine what type of repair method is appropriate for you.

The Conventional Method

In this case, an incision is made over the site of the hernia. The protruding tissue is returned to the abdominal cavity, and the sac that has formed is removed. The surgeon repairs the hole or weakness in the abdominal wall by sewing strong surrounding muscle over the defect. This is the most common method of hernia repair.

Tension-Free Mesh Technique

For this technique, an incision is made at the site of the hernia and a piece of mesh is inserted to cover the area of the abdominal wall defect without sewing together the surrounding muscles. Recovery is swift, and the likelihood of the hernia recurring is small. The mesh is safe and generally well-accepted by the body's natural tissues. However, be certain to discuss this procedure with your surgeon and understand how it will be done.

The Laparoscopic Method

A laparoscope is a long metal tube with a fiberoptic light source and a telescopic eyepiece, which is connected to a TV monitor. The scope is inserted into the abdominal cavity through a small incision and is used to view the hernia in the abdominal wall while the surgeon repairs the hernia through additional tubes that are inserted into the abdomen through separate incisions. A general anesthetic is usually required.

Some surgeons are using this technique. However, the technique is presently under evaluation, and the long-term outcome for hernias repaired using this method is currently unknown. It is important to note that this method is new, it is still being evaluated, and it is not an option for every patient. It is up to you and your surgeon to decide whether it is right for you.

Complications Are Few

As with any operation, infection and bleeding can occur. Most of the time, however, these problems are easily handled, without the need for a hospital stay. A slight chance also exists that the intestine or bladder can be injured during the operation. The formation of scar tissue is another possibility. Any infection associated with the operation will be treated with antibiotics, but otherwise such drugs are not typically used or required. It is important to note that since the laparoscopic method of hernia repair is relatively new, its complications are not as well defined as the complications that are associated with the other methods.

Recovery

As with any operation, the amount of pain that is experienced varies from patient to patient. A patient's discomfort also depends on the location and type of hernia that was repaired, as well as the technique that was used to perform the repair. Generally, you will have some difficulty walking the first few hours after the operation, and climbing stairs the first couple of days. Bathing will require care so as not to wet the incision site. Sexual activity is usually too uncomfortable to enjoy the first week or two. Your surgeon will advise you regarding heavy lifting, jogging, or doing strenuous exercise depending on the type and degree of difficulty it took to do the repair. You should be able to drive your car within a few days. Depending upon your occupation, you can expect a recovery period lasting from one to six weeks.

Proper recovery is as important as the hernia repair procedure itself. During the recovery phase, the repair takes hold. The smoother your recovery, the better the chances that your hernia will not recur. While every attempt is made to minimize any recurrence, the "perfect" repair does not exist. However, the recurrence rate over many years is small, and is estimated to be about 1–5 percent.

Reviewed by

Marvin J. Wexler, MD, FACS, FRCS, Associate Professor of Surgery, McGill University, Montreal, Quebec.

C. James Carrico, MD, FACS, Professor and Chairman, Department of Surgery, University of Texas, Dallas.

Surgery by Surgeons

A fully trained surgeon is a physician who, after medical school, has gone through years of training in an accredited residency program to learn the specialized skills of a surgeon. One good sign of a surgeon's competence is certification by a national surgical board approved by the American Board of Medical Specialties. All board-certified surgeons have satisfactorily completed an approved residency training program and have passed a rigorous specialty examination.

The letters F.A.C.S. (Fellow of the American College of Surgeons) after a surgeon's name are a further indication of a physician's qualifications. Surgeons who become Fellows of the College have passed a comprehensive evaluation of their surgical training and skills; they also have demonstrated their commitment to high standards of ethical conduct. This evaluation is conducted according to national standards that were established to ensure that patients receive the best possible surgical care.

Prepared as a public service by the American College of Surgeons.

American College of Surgeons
55 East Eric Street
Chicago, IL 60611

Chapter 25

Hirschsprung's Disease

People with Hirschsprung's disease lack the nerve cells that enable intestinal muscles to move stool through the large intestine (colon). Stool becomes trapped in the colon, filling the colon and causing it to expand to larger than normal. Hirschsprung's disease is also called megacolon. It is a congenital disease, which means a person is born with it. The disease may also be hereditary, which means a parent can pass it to a child. Hirschsprung's disease affects mainly infants and children.

Although symptoms usually begin within a few days after birth, some people don't develop them until childhood or even adulthood. In infants, the primary symptom is not passing meconium, an infant's first bowel movement, within the first 24 to 48 hours of life. Other symptoms include constipation, abdominal swelling, and vomiting. Symptoms in older children include passing small watery stools, diarrhea, and a lack of appetite.

Physicians diagnose Hirschsprung's disease through rectal manometry, a lower gastrointestinal (GI) series, and rectal biopsy. Rectal manometry involves recording pressure changes within the colon and rectum. In a lower GI series, x-rays are used to measure the width of the colon and rectum. Rectal biopsy involves removing a piece of rectal tissue to learn whether the nerve cells that control intestinal muscle contractions are present.

National Digestive Diseases Information Clearinghouse, National Institute of Diabetes and Digestive and Kidney Diseases (NIDDK), March 1998.

Colostomy is the most effective treatment for Hirschsprung's disease. In a colostomy, the surgeon removes the affected part of the colon. The top half of the remaining colon is then connected to a surgically created hole, called a stoma, on the abdomen. Stool can leave the body through this hole while the lower part of the colon heals. Later, the surgeon will reconnect the colon inside the body and close the stoma. The patient will then be able to have normal bowel movements.

For More Information

More information is available from:

American Pseudo-obstruction and Hirschsprung's Disease Society Inc.
158 Pleasant Street
North Andover, MA 01845-2797
Tel: (508) 685-4477

Pull-thru Network
4 Woody Lane
Westport, CT 06880
Tel: (203) 221-7530

Additional Information on Hirschsprung's Disease

The National Digestive Diseases Information Clearinghouse collects resource information on digestive diseases for the Combined Health Information Database (CHID). CHID is a database produced by health-related agencies of the Federal Government. This database provides titles, abstracts, and availability information for health information and health education resources.

You may access the CHID Online website and search CHID for the most up-to-date information on Hirschsprung's Disease.

Combined Health Information Database (CHID)
http://chid.nih.gov

Chapter 26

Ileostomy

A New Beginning

Now that you have, or will have an ileostomy, you are probably concerned about the changes in your life your surgery will cause. You may have some old-fashioned ideas about ostomy surgery or think there are only a few people in the world in your situation.

You should know that there are more than a million people in the United States and Canada with ostomies. They are working, playing and enjoying life just as they did before their surgery. Some are famous professional athletes, politicians and entertainers! Odds are, you have been in elevators with people with ostomies, worked with them, or played softball with them in your local league.

Think for a minute. Because an ileostomy doesn't show, it can be kept a secret if you wish. Some of your best friends may have one, but you would know only if they told you.

Some Facts about Your Surgery

An ileostomy is an opening in the abdominal wall through which digested food passes. An ileostomy may be performed when a diseased or injured colon cannot be treated successfully with medicine.

The end of the ileum (the lowest portion of the small intestine) is brought through the abdominal wall to form a stoma, usually on the lower right side of the abdomen. When you look at your stoma, you are actually looking at the lining of the intestine, which is like the lining of your cheek warm, moist and pink.

Digested food, which passes through the stoma, is collected in a device called a pouch or an appliance. The difference between today's ostomy pouches and those of the past is like the difference between night and day. Appliances today are not bulky and do not show under even the most stylish, form-fitting apparel for men and women. Whatever you wore before surgery, you can wear afterward with very few exceptions.

Pouches are odor-free and come in a variety of disposable or reusable varieties to fit your lifestyle. You are fitted for an appliance just as you are fitted for shoes or eyeglasses. Ostomy supplies are readily available at drug stores, ostomy supply houses, or through the mail.

Some procedures, called "continent ileostomies, " create an internal pouch from a patient's intestine. People with this type of ileostomy don't wear an appliance. Instead, a plastic tube is inserted into the stoma periodically during the day to drain the contents of the internal pouch. Different types of ileostomies are appropriate for different medical situations. One thing is true, however, no matter what the procedure, it is neither as difficult nor as unpleasant to live with an ileostomy as you probably imagine.

Life with an Ileostomy

You will not have to change to a new way of life, merely a new way of going to the bathroom. Adjusting to this change may seem frustrating at first, but be patient. It may take several months to complete your adjustment and reach the stage where your ileostomy is just a minor inconvenience. At first, you may find yourself spending a great amount of time in the bathroom until you become proficient with the management of your ostomy. Once you have things down pat, your routine will not take any longer than normal visits to the bathroom.

Work?

With the possible exception of jobs requiring very heavy lifting, your ileostomy should not interfere with your work. Individuals with ileostomies are successful business people, taxi drivers, welders, sales people, carpenters, teachers, etc.

Sex and Social Life?

Physically, the creation of an ileostomy usually does not affect sexual function. If there is a problem, it is almost always related to the removal of the rectum. The ileostomy itself should not interfere with pregnancy, and the risk during childbirth appears no greater than the risk for other women. An ostomy does not prevent one from dating, marriage, or having children. It will probably seem bigger and more important to you than to anyone else, including your boyfriend, girlfriend, lover, spouse, or children. Individuals with ostomies don't look different or smell bad, so your social life depends mainly on your attitude and personality.

Sports and Activities?

You can take a bath or shower with or without your pouch. Normal exposure to air or contact with soap and water will not harm your stoma. With a securely attached pouch, you can swim, camp out, climb mountains, play baseball or enjoy any other sport. (Consult your physician about heavy body-contact sports.)

You Are Not Alone

Your physician and hospital professionals are your first source of help for the many questions you have about your surgery. They can refer you to an enterostomal therapy (ET) nurse who is specially trained to help you learn to manage your stoma. They also can refer you to the United Ostomy Association (UOA) chapter in your area.

The UOA is a group of approximately 40,000 people with ostomies throughout the United States and Canada who have organized to help each other. The UOA publishes its own magazine, the *Ostomy Quarterly*, which provides updated ostomy information. It also sponsors educational conferences. Your local UOA chapter can provide an ostomy visitor who will be selected to suit your age, sex and type of ostomy. It is very reassuring to talk with someone who has already been through the things you are reading about here.

The UOA has a library of publications offering more detailed information on ostomy, particularly *Ileostomy: A Guide*. Publications cover topics such as ileostomy management, employment, sex, children and ostomy, and many others. For information on the UOA, your local chapter, or a list of UOA publications, please call or write us at the address below. Good luck, and remember, you are not alone.

United Ostomy Association
19772 MacArthur Blvd., Suite 200
Irvine, CA 92612-2405
(800) 826-0826
www.uoa.org

Chapter 27

Indigestion (Dyspepsia)

Indigestion, also known as upset stomach or dyspepsia, is a painful or burning feeling in the upper abdomen, often accompanied by nausea, abdominal bloating, belching, and sometimes vomiting.

Indigestion might be caused by a disease or an ulcer in the digestive tract, but for most people, it results from eating too much, eating too quickly, eating high-fat foods, or eating during stressful situations. Smoking, drinking too much alcohol, using medications that irritate the stomach lining, being tired, and having ongoing stress can also cause indigestion or make it worse.

Some people have persistent indigestion that is not related to any of these factors. This type of indigestion—called functional or nonulcer indigestion—is caused by a problem in how food moves through the digestive tract.

To diagnose indigestion, the doctor first rules out other problems, like ulcers. In the process of diagnosis, a person may have x-rays of the stomach and small intestine or undergo endoscopy, in which the doctor uses an instrument to look closely at the inside of the stomach.

Avoiding the foods and situations that seem to cause indigestion is the most successful way to treat it. Excess stomach acid does not cause or result from indigestion, so antacids are not an appropriate treatment, although some people report that they do help. Smokers can help relieve their indigestion by quitting smoking, or at least not

National Digestive Diseases Information Clearinghouse, National Institute of Diabetes and Digestive and Kidney Diseases (NIDDK), May 1998.

smoking right before eating. Exercising with a full stomach may cause indigestion, so scheduling exercise before a meal or at least an hour afterward might help.

To treat indigestion caused by a functional problem in the digestive tract, the doctor may prescribe medicine that affects stomach movement.

Because indigestion can be a sign of or mimic a more serious disease, people should see a doctor if they have:

- Vomiting, weight loss, or appetite loss.
- Black tarry stools or blood in vomit.
- Severe pain in the upper right abdomen.
- Discomfort unrelated to eating.
- Indigestion accompanied by shortness of breath, sweating, or pain radiating to the jaw, neck, or arm.

Additional Information on Indigestion

The National Digestive Diseases Information Clearinghouse collects resource information on digestive diseases for the Combined Health Information Database (CHID). CHID is a database produced by health-related agencies of the Federal Government. This database provides titles, abstracts, and availability information for health information and health education resources.

You may access the CHID Online website and search CHID for the most up-to-date information on Indigestion.

Combined Health Information Database (CHID)
http://chid.nih.gov

Chapter 28

Intestinal Pseudo-Obstruction

Intestinal pseudo-obstruction (false blockage) is a condition that causes symptoms like those of a bowel obstruction (blockage). But when the intestines are examined, no obstruction is found. The symptoms of intestinal pseudo-obstruction are caused by a problem in how the muscles and nerves in the intestines work.

Symptoms of pseudo-obstruction include cramps, stomach pain, nausea, vomiting, bloating, fewer bowel movements than usual, and loose stools. Over time, pseudo-obstruction can cause bacterial infections, malnutrition, and muscle problems in other parts of the body. Some people with intestinal pseudo-obstruction also have bladder problems.

Some diseases that affect muscles and nerves such as lupus erythematosus, scleroderma, or Parkinson's disease can cause symptoms of pseudo-obstruction. When a disease causes the symptoms, the condition is called secondary intestinal pseudo-obstruction. Medications that affect muscles and nerves such as opiates and antidepressants might also cause secondary pseudo-obstruction.

To diagnose the condition, the doctor will take a complete medical history, do a physical exam, and take x-rays. The main treatment is nutritional support (intravenous feeding) to prevent malnutrition, and antibiotics to treat bacterial infections. Medicine might also be given to help with intestinal muscle problems. In severe cases, surgery to remove part of the intestines might be necessary.

National Digestive Diseases Information Clearinghouse, National Institute of Diabetes and Digestive and Kidney Diseases (NIDDK), March 1998.

For More Information

More information is available from:

American Pseudo-obstruction and Hirschprung's Disease Society Inc.
158 Pleasant Street
North Andover, MA 01845-2797
tel: (508) 685-4477
e-mail: aphs@mail.tiac.net

Additional Information on Intestinal Pseudo-Obstruction

The National Digestive Diseases Information Clearinghouse collects resource information on digestive diseases for the Combined Health Information Database (CHID). CHID is a database produced by health-related agencies of the Federal Government. This database provides titles, abstracts, and availability information for health information and health education resources.

You may access the CHID Online website and search CHID for the most up-to-date information on Intestinal Pseudo-Obstruction

Combined Health Information Database (CHID)
http://chid.nih.gov

Chapter 29

Irritable Bowel Syndrome

Questions and Answers about Irritable Bowel Syndrome

What Is Irritable Bowel Syndrome?

Irritable bowel syndrome (IBS) is a common disorder of the intestines that leads to crampy pain, gassiness, bloating, and changes in bowel habits. Some people with IBS have constipation (difficult or infrequent bowel movements); others have diarrhea (frequent loose stools, often with an urgent need to move the bowels); and some people experience both. Sometimes the person with IBS has a crampy urge to move the bowels but cannot do so.

Through the years, IBS has been called by many names—colitis, mucous colitis, spastic colon, spastic bowel, and functional bowel disease. Most of these terms are inaccurate. Colitis, for instance, means inflammation of the large intestine (colon). IBS, however, does not cause inflammation and should not be confused with another disorder, ulcerative colitis.

The cause of IBS is not known, and as yet there is no cure. Doctors call it a functional disorder because there is no sign of disease when the colon is examined. IBS causes a great deal of discomfort and distress, but it does not cause permanent harm to the intestines and does not lead to intestinal bleeding of the bowel or to a serious disease

National Institute of Diabetes and Digestive and Kidney Diseases (NIDDK), National Institute of Health, NIH Pub. No. 97-693, 1992.

such as cancer. Often IBS is just a mild annoyance, but for some people it can be disabling. They may be unable to go to social events, to go out to a job, or to travel even short distances. Most people with IBS, however, are able to control their symptoms through medications prescribed by their physicians, diet, and stress management.

What Causes IBS?

The colon, which is about 6 feet long, connects the small intestine with the rectum and anus. The major function of the colon is to absorb water and salts from digestive products that enter from the small intestine. Two quarts of liquid matter enter the colon from the small intestine each day. This material may remain there for several days until most of the fluid and salts are absorbed into the body. The stool then passes through the colon by a pattern of movements to the left side of the colon, where it is stored until a bowel movement occurs.

Colon motility (contraction of intestinal muscles and movement of its contents) is controlled by nerves and hormones and by electrical activity in the colon muscle. The electrical activity serves as a "pacemaker" similar to the mechanism that controls heart function.

Movements of the colon propel the contents slowly back and forth but mainly toward the rectum. A few times each day strong muscle contractions move down the colon pushing fecal material ahead of them. Some of these strong contractions result in a bowel movement.

Because doctors have been unable to find an organic cause, IBS often has been thought to be caused by emotional conflict or stress. While stress may worsen IBS symptoms, research suggests that other factors also are important. Researchers have found that the colon muscle of a person with IBS begins to spasm after only mild stimulation. The person with IBS seems to have a colon that is more sensitive and reactive than usual, so it responds strongly to stimuli that would not bother most people.

Ordinary events such as eating and distention from gas or other material in the colon can cause the colon to overreact in the person with IBS. Certain medicines and foods may trigger spasms in some people. Sometimes the spasm delays the passage of stool, leading to constipation. Chocolate, milk products, or large amounts of alcohol are frequent offenders. Caffeine causes loose stools in many people, but it is more likely to affect those with IBS. Researchers also have found that women with IBS may have more symptoms during their menstrual periods, suggesting that reproductive hormones can increase IBS symptoms.

What Are the Symptoms of IBS?

If you are concerned about IBS, it is important to realize that normal bowel function varies from person to person. Normal bowel movements range from as many as three stools a day to as few as three a week. A normal movement is one that is formed but not hard, contains no blood, and is passed without cramps or pain.

People with IBS, on the other hand, usually have crampy abdominal pain with painful constipation or diarrhea. In some people, constipation and diarrhea alternate. Sometimes people with IBS pass mucus with their bowel movements. Bleeding, fever, weight loss, and persistent severe pain are not symptoms of IBS but may indicate other problems.

How Is IBS Diagnosed?

IBS usually is diagnosed after doctors exclude the presence of disease. To get to that point, the doctor will take a complete medical history that includes a careful description of symptoms. A physical examination and laboratory tests will be done. A stool sample will be tested for evidence of bleeding. The doctor also may do diagnostic procedures such as x-rays or endoscopy (viewing the colon through a flexible tube inserted through the anus) to find out if there is disease.

How Do Diet and Stress Affect IBS?

The potential for abnormal function of the colon is always present in people with IBS, but a trigger also must be present to cause symptoms. The most likely culprits seem to be diet and emotional stress. Many people report that their symptoms occur following a meal or when they are under stress. No one is sure why this happens, but scientists have some clues.

Eating causes contractions of the colon. Normally, this response may cause an urge to have a bowel movement within 30 to 60 minutes after a meal. In people with IBS, the urge may come sooner with cramps and diarrhea.

The strength of the response is often related to the number of calories in a meal and especially the amount of fat in a meal. Fat in any form (animal or vegetable) is a strong stimulus of colonic contractions after a meal. Many foods contain fat, especially meats of all kinds, poultry skin, whole milk, cream, cheese, butter, vegetable oil, margarine, shortening, avocados, and whipped toppings.

Stress also stimulates colonic spasm in people with IBS. This process is not completely understood, but scientists point out that the colon is controlled partly by the nervous system. Stress reduction (relaxation) training or counseling and support help relieve IBS symptoms in some people. However, doctors are quick to note that this does not mean IBS is the result of a personality disorder. IBS is at least partly a disorder of colon motility.

How Does a Good Diet Help IBS?

For many people, eating a proper diet lessens IBS symptoms. Before changing your diet, it is a good idea to keep a journal noting which foods seem to cause distress. Discuss your findings with your doctor. You also may want to consult a registered dietitian, who can help you make changes in your diet. For instance, if dairy products cause your symptoms to flare up, you can try eating less of those foods. Yogurt might be tolerated better because it contains organisms that supply lactase, the enzyme needed to digest lactose, the sugar found in milk products. Because dairy products are an important source of calcium and other nutrients that your body needs, be sure to get adequate nutrients in the foods that you substitute.

Dietary fiber may lessen IBS symptoms in many cases. Whole grain breads and cereals, beans, fruits, and vegetables are good sources of fiber. Consult your doctor before using an over-the-counter fiber supplement. High-fiber diets keep the colon mildly distended, which may help to prevent spasms from developing. Some forms of fiber also keep water in the stools, thereby preventing hard stools that are difficult to pass. Doctors usually recommend that you eat just enough fiber so that you have soft, easily passed, and painless bowel movements. High-fiber diets may cause gas and bloating, but within a few weeks, these symptoms often go away as your body adjusts to the diet.

Large meals can cause cramping and diarrhea in people with IBS. Symptoms may be eased if you eat smaller meals more often or just eat smaller portions. This should help, especially if your meals are low in fat and high in carbohydrates such as pasta, rice, whole-grain breads and cereals, fruits, and vegetables.

Can Medicines Relieve IBS Symptoms?

There is no standard way of treating IBS. Your doctor may prescribe fiber supplements or occasional laxatives if you are constipated.

Some doctors prescribe drugs that control colon muscle spasms, drugs that slow the movement of food through the digestive system, or tranquilizers, all of which may relieve symptoms. Antidepressant drugs also are used sometimes in patients who are depressed.

It is important to follow the physician's instructions when taking IBS medications—particularly laxatives, which can be habit forming if not used carefully.

Is IBS Linked to Other Diseases?

IBS has not been shown to lead to any serious, organic diseases. No link has been established between IBS and inflammatory bowel diseases such as Crohn's disease or ulcerative colitis. IBS does not lead to cancer. Some patients have a more severe form of IBS, and the pain and diarrhea may cause them to withdraw from normal activities. These patients need to work with their physicians to find the best combination of medicine, diet, counseling, and support to control their symptoms.

Additional Readings

- Scanlon, D, Becnel, B. *Wellness Book of IBS*. New York: St. Martin's Press, 1989. Practical patient's guide to coping with IBS written by a registered dietitian. Available in libraries and bookstores.

- Shimberg, E. *Relief From IBS*. New York: M. Evans and Company, 1988. Practical book for patients offers information about IBS symptoms, diet, treatment, and self-care. Available in libraries and bookstores.

- Steinhart, MJ. Irritable bowel syndrome: How to relieve symptoms enough to improve daily function. *Postgraduate Medicine* 1992; 91(6): 315-321. Article for primary care physicians includes information about relief of IBS symptoms. Available in medical and university libraries.

- Thompson, WG. *Gut reactions: Understanding symptoms of the digestive tract*. New York: Plenum Publishing Corp.,1989. Clear, concise book by a digestive diseases specialist gives advice about diagnosis, diet, and treatment of IBS. Available in libraries and bookstores.

Chapter 30

Irritable Bowel Syndrome in Children

Irritable bowel syndrome (IBS) is a digestive disorder that causes abdominal pain, bloating, gas, diarrhea, and constipation—or some combination of these problems. IBS affects people of all ages, including children.

IBS is classified as a functional disorder because it is caused by a problem in how the intestines, or bowels, work. People with IBS tend to have overly sensitive intestines that have muscle spasms in response to food, gas, and sometimes stress. These spasms may cause pain, diarrhea, and constipation.

In children, IBS tends to be either diarrhea-predominant or pain-predominant. Diarrhea-predominant IBS is most common in children under age 3. The diarrhea is usually painless and alternates with bouts of constipation. These children usually have fewer than five stools a day, and the stools tend to be watery and soft. Pain-predominant IBS mainly affects children over age 5. In the younger children the pain tends to occur around the navel area, and in older children, in the lower left part of the abdomen. The pain is crampy and gets worse with eating and better after passing stool or gas.

In addition to the symptoms described above, children with IBS may also have headache, nausea, or mucus in the stool. Weight loss may occur if a child eats less to try to avoid pain. Some children first develop symptoms after a stressful event, such as teething, a bout with

National Digestive Diseases Information Clearinghouse, National Institute of Diabetes and Digestive and Kidney Diseases (NIDDK), April 1998.

the flu, school problems, or problems at home. Stress does not cause IBS, but it can trigger symptoms.

To diagnose IBS, the doctor will ask questions about symptoms and examine the child to rule out the possibility of more serious problems or diseases. IBS is not a disease—it is a syndrome, or group of symptoms that occur together. It does not damage the intestine, so if the physical exam and other tests show no sign of disease or damage, the doctor may diagnose IBS.

In children, IBS is treated mainly through changes in diet—eating more fiber and less fat to help prevent spasms—and through bowel training to teach the child to empty the bowels at regular, specific times during the day. Medications like laxatives are rarely prescribed because children are more susceptible to addiction than adults. When laxatives are necessary, parents must follow the doctor's instructions carefully. Learning stress management techniques may help some children.

For More Information

More information is available from:

International Foundation for Functional Gastrointestinal Disorders
P.O. Box 17864
Milwaukee, WI 53217
Tel: (414) 241-9479
Web site: http://www.execpc.com/iffgd

Additional Information on Irritable Bowel Syndrome in Children

The National Digestive Diseases Information Clearinghouse collects resource information on digestive diseases for the Combined Health Information Database (CHID). CHID is a database produced by health-related agencies of the Federal Government. This database provides titles, abstracts, and availability information for health information and health education resources.

You may access the CHID Online website and search CHID for the most up-to-date information on Irritable Bowel Syndrome in Children.

Combined Health Information Database (CHID)
http://chid.nih.gov

Chapter 31

Lactose Intolerance

What Is Lactose Intolerance?

Lactose intolerance is the inability to digest significant amounts of lactose, the predominant sugar of milk. This inability results from a shortage of the enzyme lactase, which is normally produced by the cells that line the small intestine. Lactase breaks down milk sugar into simpler forms that can then be absorbed into the bloodstream. When there is not enough lactase to digest the amount of lactose consumed, the results, although not usually dangerous, may be very distressing. While not all persons deficient in lactase have symptoms, those who do are considered to be lactose intolerant.

Common symptoms include nausea, cramps, bloating, gas, and diarrhea, which begin about 30 minutes to 2 hours after eating or drinking foods containing lactose. The severity of symptoms varies depending on the amount of lactose each individual can tolerate.

Some causes of lactose intolerance are well known. For instance, certain digestive diseases and injuries to the small intestine can reduce the amount of enzymes produced. In rare cases, children are born without the ability to produce lactase. For most people, though, lactase deficiency is a condition that develops naturally over time. After about the age of 2 years, the body begins to produce less lactase. However, many people may not experience symptoms until they are much older.

National Institute of Diabetes and Digestive and Kidney Diseases (NIDDK), NIH Pub. No. 98-2751, updated November 1998.

Between 30 and 50 million Americans are lactose intolerant. Certain ethnic and racial populations are more widely affected than others. As many as 75 percent of all African-Americans and Native Americans and 90 percent of Asian-Americans are lactose intolerant. The condition is least common among persons of northern European descent.

How Is Lactose Intolerance Diagnosed?

The most common tests used to measure the absorption of lactose in the digestive system are the lactose tolerance test, the hydrogen breath test, and the stool acidity test. These tests are performed on an outpatient basis at a hospital, clinic, or doctor's office.

The lactose tolerance test begins with the individual fasting (not eating) before the test and then drinking a liquid that contains lactose. Several blood samples are taken over a 2-hour period to measure the person's blood glucose (blood sugar) level, which indicates how well the body is able to digest lactose.

Normally, when lactose reaches the digestive system, the lactase enzyme breaks down lactase into glucose and galactose. The liver then changes the galactose into glucose, which enters the bloodstream and raises the person's blood glucose level. If lactose is incompletely broken down the blood glucose level does not rise, and a diagnosis of lactose intolerance is confirmed.

The hydrogen breath test measures the amount of hydrogen in the breath. Normally, very little hydrogen is detectable in the breath. However, undigested lactose in the colon is fermented by bacteria, and various gases, including hydrogen, are produced. The hydrogen is absorbed from the intestines, carried through the bloodstream to the lungs, and exhaled. In the test, the patient drinks a lactose-loaded beverage, and the breath is analyzed at regular intervals. Raised levels of hydrogen in the breath indicate improper digestion of lactose. Certain foods, medications, and cigarettes can affect the test's accuracy and should be avoided before taking the test. This test is available for children and adults.

The lactose tolerance and hydrogen breath tests are not given to infants and very young children who are suspected of having lactose intolerance. A large lactose load may be dangerous for very young individuals because they are more prone to dehydration that can result from diarrhea caused by the lactose. If a baby or young child is experiencing symptoms of lactose intolerance, many pediatricians simply recommend changing from cow's milk to soy formula and waiting for symptoms to abate.

If necessary, a stool acidity test, which measures the amount of acid in the stool, may be given to infants and young children. Undigested lactose fermented by bacteria in the colon creates lactic acid and other short-chain fatty acids that can be detected in a stool sample. In addition, glucose may be present in the sample as a result of unabsorbed lactose in the colon.

How Is Lactose Intolerance Treated?

Fortunately, lactose intolerance is relatively easy to treat. No treatment exists to improve the body's ability to produce lactase, but symptoms can be controlled through diet.

Young children with lactase deficiency should not eat any foods containing lactose. Most older children and adults need not avoid lactose completely, but individuals differ in the amounts of lactose they can handle. For example, one person may suffer symptoms after drinking a small glass of milk, while another can drink one glass but not two. Others may be able to manage ice cream and aged cheeses, such as cheddar and Swiss but not other dairy products. Dietary control of lactose intolerance depends on each person's learning through trial and error how much lactose he or she can handle.

For those who react to very small amounts of lactose or have trouble limiting their intake of foods that contain lactose, lactase enzymes are available without a prescription. One form is a liquid for use with milk. A few drops are added to a quart of milk, and after 24 hours in the refrigerator, the lactose content is reduced by 70 percent. The process works faster if the milk is heated first, and adding a double amount of lactase liquid produces milk that is 90 percent lactose free. A more recent development is a chewable lactase enzyme tablet that helps people digest solid foods that contain lactose. Three to six tablets are taken just before a meal or snack.

Lactose-reduced milk and other products are available at many supermarkets. The milk contains all of the nutrients found in regular milk and remains fresh for about the same length of time or longer if it is super-pasteurized.

How Is Nutrition Balanced?

Milk and other dairy products are a major source of nutrients in the American diet. The most important of these nutrients is calcium. Calcium is essential for the growth and repair of bones throughout life. In the middle and later years, a shortage of calcium may lead to thin, fragile bones that break easily (a condition called osteoporosis). A concern, then, for both children and adults with lactose intolerance, is getting enough calcium in a diet that includes little or no milk.

In 1997, the Institute of Medicine released a report recommending new requirements for daily calcium intake. How much calcium a person needs to maintain good health varies by age group. Recommendations from the report are show in Table 31.1.

Table 31.1. Daily Calcium Intake Recommendations

Age group	Amount of calcium to consume daily in milligrams (mg)
0-6 months	210 mg
6-12 months	270 mg
1-3 years	500 mg
4-8 years	800 mg
9-18 years	1,300 mg
19-50 years	1,000 mg
51-70 years	1,200 mg

Also, pregnant and nursing women under 19 need 1,300 mg daily, while pregnant and nursing women over 19 need 1,000 mg.

In planning meals, making sure that each day's diet includes enough calcium is important, even if the diet does not contain dairy products. Many nondairy foods are high in calcium. Green vegetables, such as broccoli and kale, and fish with soft, edible bones, such as salmon and sardines, are excellent sources of calcium. To help in planning a high-calcium and low-lactose diet, Table 31.2 lists some common foods that are good sources of dietary calcium and shows about how much lactose the foods contain.

Recent research shows that yogurt with active cultures may be a good source of calcium for many people with lactose intolerance, even though it is fairly high in lactose. Evidence shows that the bacterial cultures used in making yogurt produce some of the lactase enzyme required for proper digestion.

Clearly, many foods can provide the calcium and other nutrients the body needs, even when intake of milk and dairy products is limited.

Table 31.2. Calcium and Lactose in Common Foods

Food	Calcium Content*	Lactose Content**
Vegetables		
Brocolli (cooked), 1 cup	94-177 mg	0
Chinese cabbage (bok choy, cooked), 1 cup	158 mg	0
Collard greens (cooked), 1 cup	148-357 mg	0
Kale (cooked), 1 cup	94-179 mg	0
Turnip greens (cooked), 1 cup	194-249 mg	0
Dairy Products		
Ice cream/Ice milk, 8 oz	176 mg	6-7 g
Milk (whole, low-fat, skim, buttermilk) 8 oz	291-316 mg	12-13 g
Processed cheese, 1 oz	159-219 mg	2-3 g
Sour cream, 4 oz	134 mg	4-5 g
Yogurt (plain), 8 oz	274-415 mg	12-13 g
Fish/Seafood		
Oysters (raw), 1 cup	226 mg	0
Salmon with bones (canned), 3 oz	167 mg	0
Sardines, 3 oz	371 mg	0
Shrimp (canned), 3 oz	98 mg	0
Other		
Molasses, 2 tbsp	274 mg	0
Tofu (processed with calcium salts), 3 oz	225 mg	0

* Nutritive Value of Foods. Values vary with methods of processing and preparation.

**Derived from *Lactose Intolerance: A Resource Including Recipes*, Food Sensitivity Series, American Dietetic Association, 1991.

However, factors other than calcium and lactose content should be kept in mind when planning a diet. Some vegetables that are high in calcium (Swiss chard, spinach, and rhubarb, for instance) are not listed in Table 31.2 because the body cannot use their calcium content. They contain substances called oxalates, which stop calcium absorption. Calcium is absorbed and used only when there is enough vitamin D in the body. A balanced diet should provide an adequate supply of vitamin D. Sources of vitamin D include eggs and liver. However, sunlight helps the body naturally absorb or synthesize vitamin D, and with enough exposure to the sun, food sources may not be necessary.

Some people with lactose intolerance may think they are not getting enough calcium and vitamin D in their diet. Consultation with a doctor or dietitian may be helpful in deciding whether any dietary supplements are needed. Taking vitamins or minerals of the wrong kind or in the wrong amounts can be harmful. A dietitian can help in planning meals that will provide the most nutrients with the least chance of causing discomfort.

What Is Hidden Lactose?

Although milk and foods made from milk are the only natural sources, lactose is often added to prepared foods. People with very low tolerance for lactose should know about the many food products that may contain lactose, even in small amounts. Food products that may contain lactose include:

- Bread and other baked goods
- Processed breakfast cereals
- Instant potatoes, soups, and breakfast drinks
- Margarine
- Lunch meats (other than kosher)
- Salad dressings
- Candies and other snacks
- Mixes for pancakes, biscuits, and cookies

Some products labeled nondairy, such as powdered coffee creamer and whipped toppings, may also include ingredients that are derived from milk and therefore contain lactose.

Smart shoppers learn to read food labels with care, looking not only for milk and lactose among the contents but also for such words as whey, curds, milk by-products, dry milk solids, and nonfat dry milk powder. If any of these are listed on a label, the item contains lactose.

In addition, lactose is used as the base for more than 20 percent of prescription drugs and about 6 percent of over-the-counter medicines. Many types of birth control pills, for example, contain lactose, as do some tablets for stomach acid and gas. However, these products typically affect only people with severe lactose intolerance.

Summary

Even though lactose intolerance is widespread, it need not pose a serious threat to good health. People who have trouble digesting lactose can learn which dairy products and other foods they can eat without discomfort and which ones they should avoid. Many will be able to enjoy milk, ice cream, and other such products if they take them in small amounts or eat other food at the same time. Others can use lactase liquid or tablets to help digest the lactose. Even older women at risk for osteoporosis and growing children who must avoid milk and foods made with milk can meet most of their special dietary needs by eating greens, fish, and other calcium-rich foods that are free of lactose. A carefully chosen diet (with calcium supplements if the doctor or dietitian recommends them) is the key to reducing symptoms and protecting future health.

For More Information

National Digestive Diseases Information Clearinghouse
2 Information Way
Bethesda, MD 20892-3570
E-mail: nddic@info.niddk.nih.gov

The National Digestive Diseases Information Clearinghouse (NDDIC) is a service of the National Institute of Diabetes and Digestive and Kidney Diseases (NIDDK). NIDDK is part of the National Institutes of Health under the U.S. Department of Health and Human Services. Established in 1980, the clearinghouse provides information about digestive diseases to people with digestive disorders and to their families, health care professionals, and the public. NDDIC answers inquiries; develops, reviews, and distributes publications; and works closely with professional and patient organizations and Government agencies to coordinate resources about digestive diseases.

Publications produced by the clearinghouse are reviewed carefully for scientific accuracy, content, and readability.

Chapter 32

Ménétrier's Disease

Ménétrier's disease causes giant folds of tissue to grow in the wall of the stomach. The tissue may be inflamed and may contain ulcers. The disease also causes glands in the stomach to waste away and interferes with the body's absorption of a protein called albumin. Ménétrier's disease increases a person's risk of stomach cancer. People who have this rare, chronic disease are usually men between ages 30 and 60. The cause of the disease is unknown.

Symptoms include pain or discomfort and tenderness in the top middle part of the abdomen, loss of appetite, nausea, vomiting, diarrhea, vomiting blood, swelling in the abdomen, and ulcer-like pain after eating.

Ménétrier's disease is diagnosed through x-rays, endoscopy, and biopsy of stomach tissue. Endoscopy involves looking at the inside of the stomach using a long, lighted tube that is inserted through the mouth. Biopsy involves removing a tiny piece of stomach tissue to examine under the microscope for signs of disease.

Treatment may include medications to relieve ulcer symptoms and treat inflammation, and a high-protein diet. Part or all of the stomach may need to be removed if the disease is severe.

For More Information

Information is available from:

National Digestive Diseases Information Clearinghouse, National Institute of Diabetes and Digestive and Kidney Diseases (NIDDK), March 1998.

National Organization for Rare Disorders Inc.
P.O. Box 8923
New Fairfield, CT 06812-8923
Tel: (800) 999-6673 or (203) 746-6518

Additional Information on Ménétrier's Disease

The National Digestive Diseases Information Clearinghouse collects resource information on digestive diseases for the Combined Health Information Database (CHID). CHID is a database produced by health-related agencies of the Federal Government. This database provides titles, abstracts, and availability information for health information and health education resources.

You may access the CHID Online website and search CHID for the most up-to-date information on Ménétrier's Disease.

Combined Health Information Database (CHID)
http://chid.nih.gov

Chapter 33

Rapid Gastric Emptying

Rapid gastric emptying, or dumping syndrome, happens when the lower end of the small intestine (jejunum) fills too quickly with undigested food from the stomach. "Early" dumping begins during or right after a meal. Symptoms of early dumping include nausea, vomiting, bloating, diarrhea, and shortness of breath. "Late" dumping happens 1 to 3 hours after eating. Symptoms of late dumping include weakness, sweating, and dizziness. Many people have both types.

Stomach surgery is the main cause of dumping syndrome because surgery may damage the system that controls digestion. Patients with Zollinger-Ellison syndrome may also have dumping syndrome. (Zollinger-Ellison syndrome is a rare disorder involving extreme peptic ulcer disease and gastrin-secreting tumors in the pancreas.)

Doctors diagnose dumping syndrome through blood tests. Treatment includes changes in eating habits and medication. People who have dumping syndrome need to eat several small meals a day that are low in carbohydrates and should drink liquids between meals, not with them. People with severe cases take medicine to slow their digestion.

Additional Information on Rapid Gastric Emptying

The National Digestive Diseases Information Clearinghouse collects resource information on digestive diseases for the Combined

National Digestive Diseases Information Clearinghouse, National Institute of Diabetes and Digestive and Kidney Diseases (NIDDK), March 1998.

Health Information Database (CHID). CHID is a database produced by health-related agencies of the Federal Government. This database provides titles, abstracts, and availability information for health information and health education resources.

You may access the CHID Online website and search CHID for the most up-to-date information on Rapid Gastric Emptying.

Combined Health Information Database (CHID)
http://chid.nih.gov

Chapter 34

Short Bowel Syndrome

Short bowel syndrome is a group of problems affecting people who have had half or more of their small intestine removed. The most common reason for removing part of the small intestine is to treat Crohn's disease.

Diarrhea is the main symptom of short bowel syndrome. Other symptoms include cramping, bloating, and heartburn. Many people with short bowel syndrome are malnourished because their remaining small intestine is unable to absorb enough water, vitamins, and other nutrients from food. They may also become dehydrated, which can be life threatening. Problems associated with dehydration and malnutrition include weakness, fatigue, depression, weight loss, bacterial infections, and food sensitivities.

Short bowel syndrome is treated through changes in diet, intravenous feeding, vitamin and mineral supplements, and medicine to relieve symptoms.

Additional Information on Short Bowel Syndrome

The National Digestive Diseases Information Clearinghouse collects resource information on digestive diseases for the Combined Health Information Database (CHID). CHID is a database produced by health-related agencies of the Federal Government. This database

National Digestive Diseases Information Clearinghouse, National Institute of Diabetes and Digestive and Kidney Diseases (NIDDK), March 1998.

provides titles, abstracts, and availability information for health information and health education resources.

You may access the CHID Online website and search CHID for the most up-to-date information on Short Bowel Syndrome.

Combined Health Information Database (CHID)
http://chid.nih.gov

Chapter 35

Ulcerative Colitis

Ulcerative colitis is a disease that causes inflammation and sores, called ulcers, in the top layers of the lining of the large intestine. The inflammation usually occurs in the rectum and lower part of the colon, but it may affect the entire colon. Ulcerative colitis rarely affects the small intestine except for the lower section, called the ileum. Ulcerative colitis may also be called colitis, ileitis, or proctitis.

The inflammation makes the colon empty frequently, causing diarrhea. Ulcers form in places where the inflammation has killed colon lining cells; the ulcers bleed and produce pus and mucus.

Ulcerative colitis is an inflammatory bowel disease (IBD), the general name for diseases that cause inflammation in the intestines. Ulcerative colitis can be difficult to diagnose because its symptoms are similar to other intestinal disorders such as irritable bowel syndrome and to another type of IBD called Crohn's disease. Crohn's disease differs from ulcerative colitis because it causes inflammation deeper within the intestinal wall. Crohn's disease usually occurs in the small intestine, but it can also occur in the mouth, esophagus, stomach, duodenum, large intestine, appendix, and anus.

Ulcerative colitis occurs most often in people ages 15 to 40, although children and older people sometimes develop the disease. Ulcerative colitis affects men and women equally and appears to run in some families.

National Institute of Diabetes and Digestive and Kidney Diseases (NIDDK), National Institutes of Health, NIH Pub. No. 98-1597, April 1998.

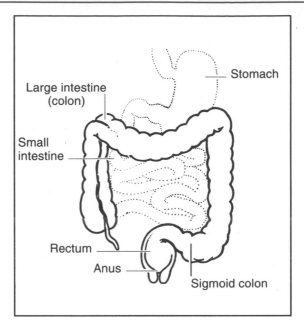

Figure 35.1. Colon.

What Causes Ulcerative Colitis?

Theories about what causes ulcerative colitis abound, but none have been proven. The most popular theory is that the body's immune system reacts to a virus or a bacterium by causing ongoing inflammation in the intestinal wall.

People with ulcerative colitis have abnormalities of the immune system, but doctors do not know whether these abnormalities are a cause or a result of the disease. Ulcerative colitis is not caused by emotional distress or sensitivity to certain foods or food products, but these factors may trigger symptoms in some people.

What Are the Symptoms of Ulcerative Colitis?

The most common symptoms of ulcerative colitis are abdominal pain and bloody diarrhea. Patients also may experience:

- Fatigue.
- Weight loss.
- Loss of appetite.

- Rectal bleeding.
- Loss of body fluids and nutrients.

About half of patients have mild symptoms. Others suffer frequent fever, bloody diarrhea, nausea, and severe abdominal cramps. Ulcerative colitis may also cause problems such as arthritis, inflammation of the eye, liver disease (fatty liver, hepatitis, cirrhosis, and primary sclerosing cholangitis), osteoporosis, skin rashes, anemia, and kidney stones. No one knows for sure why problems occur outside the colon. Scientists think these complications may occur when the immune system triggers inflammation in other parts of the body. These problems are usually mild and go away when the colitis is treated.

How Is Ulcerative Colitis Diagnosed?

A thorough physical exam and a series of tests may be required to diagnose ulcerative colitis.

Blood tests may be done to check for anemia, which could indicate bleeding in the colon or rectum. Blood tests may also uncover a high white blood cell count, which is a sign of inflammation somewhere in the body. By testing a stool sample, the doctor can tell if there is bleeding or infection in the colon or rectum.

The doctor may do a colonoscopy. For this test, the doctor inserts an endoscope—a long, flexible, lighted tube connected to a computer and TV monitor—into the anus to see the inside of the colon and rectum. The doctor will be able to see any inflammation, bleeding, or ulcers on the colon wall. During the exam, the doctor may do a biopsy, which involves taking a sample of tissue from the lining of the colon to view with a microscope. A barium enema x-ray of the colon may also be required. This procedure involves filling the colon with barium, a chalky white solution. The barium shows up white on x-ray film, allowing the doctor a clear view of the colon, including any ulcers or other abnormalities that might be there.

What Is the Treatment for Ulcerative Colitis?

Treatment for ulcerative colitis depends on the seriousness of the disease. Most people are treated with medication. In severe cases, a patient may need surgery to remove the diseased colon. Surgery is the only cure for ulcerative colitis.

Some people whose symptoms are triggered by certain foods are able to control the symptoms by avoiding foods that upset their intestines, like highly seasoned foods or milk sugar (lactose). Each person may experience ulcerative colitis differently, so treatment is adjusted for each individual. Emotional and psychological support is important.

Some people have remissions—periods when the symptoms go away—that last for months or even years. However, most patients' symptoms eventually return. This changing pattern of the disease means one cannot always tell when a treatment has helped.

Someone with ulcerative colitis may need medical care for some time, with regular doctor visits to monitor the condition.

Drug Therapy

Most patients with mild or moderate disease are first treated with 5-ASA agents, a combination of the drugs sulfonamide, sulfapyridine, and salicylate that helps control inflammation. Sulfasalazine is the most commonly used of these drugs. Sulfasalazine can be used for as long as needed and can be given along with other drugs. Patients who do not do well on sulfasalazine may respond to newer 5-ASA agents. Possible side effects of 5-ASA preparations include nausea, vomiting, heartburn, diarrhea, and headache.

People with severe disease and those who do not respond to mesalamine preparations may be treated with corticosteroids. Prednisone and hydrocortisone are two corticosteroids used to reduce inflammation. They can be given orally, intravenously, through an enema, or in a suppository, depending on the location of the inflammation. Corticosteroids can cause side effects such as weight gain, acne, facial hair, hypertension, mood swings, and increased risk of infection, so doctors carefully watch patients taking these drugs.

Other drugs may be given to relax the patient or to relieve pain, diarrhea, or infection.

Occasionally, symptoms are severe enough that the person must be hospitalized. For example, a person may have severe bleeding or severe diarrhea that causes dehydration. In such cases the doctor will try to stop diarrhea and loss of blood, fluids, and mineral salts. The patient may need a special diet, feeding through a vein, medications, or sometimes surgery.

Surgery

About 25 percent to 40 percent of ulcerative colitis patients must eventually have their colons removed because of massive bleeding, severe illness, rupture of the colon, or risk of cancer. Sometimes the doctor will recommend removing the colon if medical treatment fails or if the side effects of corticosteroids or other drugs threaten the patient's health.

One of several surgeries may be done. The most common surgery is a proctocolectomy with ileostomy, which is done in two stages. In the proctocolectomy, the surgeon removes the colon and rectum. In the ileostomy, the surgeon creates a small opening in the abdomen, called a stoma, and attaches the end of the small intestine, called the ileum, to it. This type of ileostomy is called a Brooke ileostomy. Waste will travel through the small intestine and exit the body through the stoma. The stoma is about the size of a quarter and is usually located in the lower right part of the abdomen near the beltline. A pouch is worn over the opening to collect waste, and the patient empties the pouch as needed.

An alternative to the Brooke ileostomy is the continent ileostomy. In this operation, the surgeon uses the ileum to create a pouch inside the lower abdomen. Waste empties into this pouch, and the patient drains the pouch by inserting a tube into it through a small, leakproof opening in his or her side. The patient must wear an external pouch for only the first few months after the operation. Possible complications of the continent ileostomy include malfunction of the leakproof opening, which requires surgical repair, and inflammation of the pouch (pouchitis), which is treated with antibiotics.

An ileoanal anastomosis, or pull-through operation, allows the patient to have normal bowel movements because it preserves part of the rectum. This procedure is becoming increasingly common for ulcerative colitis. In this operation, the surgeon removes the diseased part of the colon and the inside of the rectum, leaving the outer muscles of the rectum. The surgeon then attaches the ileum to the inside of the rectum and the anus, creating a pouch. Waste is stored in the pouch and passed through the anus in the usual manner. Bowel movements may be more frequent and watery than usual. Pouchitis is a possible complication of this procedure.

Not every operation is appropriate for every person. Which surgery to have depends on the severity of the disease and the patient's needs, expectations, and lifestyle. People faced with this decision should get as much information as possible by talking to their doctors, to nurses who work with colon surgery patients (enterostomal therapists), and to other colon surgery patients. Patient advocacy organizations can direct people to support groups and other information resources. (See Resources for the names of such organizations.)

221

Most people with ulcerative colitis will never need to have surgery. If surgery ever does become necessary, however, some people find comfort in knowing that after the surgery, the colitis is cured and most people go on to live normal, active lives.

Research

Researchers are always looking for new treatments for ulcerative colitis. Several drugs are being tested to see whether they might be useful in treating the disease:

Budesonide. A corticosteroid called budesonide may be nearly as effective as prednisone in treating mild ulcerative colitis, and it has fewer side effects.

Cyclosporine. Cyclosporine, a drug that suppresses the immune system, may be a promising treatment for people who do not respond to 5-ASA preparations or corticosteroids.

Nicotine. In an early study, symptoms improved in some patients who were given nicotine through a patch or an enema. (Using nicotine as treatment is still experimental—the findings do not mean that people should go out and buy nicotine patches or start smoking.)

Heparin. Researchers overseas are examining whether the anticoagulant heparin can help control colitis by preventing blood clots.

Is Colon Cancer a Concern?

About 5 percent of people with ulcerative colitis develop colon cancer. The risk of cancer increases with the duration and the extent of involvement of the colon. For example, if only the lower colon and rectum are involved, the risk of cancer is not higher than normal. However, if the entire colon is involved, the risk of cancer may be as great as 32 times the normal rate.

Sometimes precancerous changes occur in the cells lining the colon. These changes are called "dysplasia." People who have dysplasia are more likely to develop cancer than those who do not. (Doctors look for signs of dysplasia when doing a colonoscopy and when examining tissue removed during the test.)

According to 1997 guidelines on screening for colon cancer, people who have had IBD throughout their colon for at least 8 years and those who have had IBD in only the left colon for at least 15 years should have a colonoscopy every 1 to 2 years to check for dysplasia. Such screening has not been proven to reduce the risk of colon cancer, but it may help identify cancer early should it develop. (These guidelines were produced by an independent expert panel and endorsed by numerous organizations, including the American Cancer Society, American College of Gastroenterology, American Society of Colon and Rectal Surgeons, and the Crohn's & Colitis Foundation of America Inc., among others.)

Resources

Crohn's & Colitis Foundation of America Inc.
386 Park Avenue South, 17th floor
New York, NY 10016-8804
Tel: (800) 932-2423 or (212) 685-3440
E-mail: info@ccfa.org
Home page: http://www.ccfa.org

Pediatric Crohn's & Colitis Association Inc.
P.O. Box 188
Newton, MA 02168
Tel: (617) 489-5854

Pull-thru Network
4 Woody Lane
Westport, CT 06880
Tel: (203) 221-7530
E-mail: pullthrunw@aol.com
Home page: http://members.aol.com/pullthrunw/Pullthru.html

Reach Out for Youth with Ileitis and Colitis Inc.
15 Chemung Place
Jericho, NY 11753
Tel: (516) 822-8010

United Ostomy Association
36 Executive Park, Suite 120
Irvine, CA 92714
Tel: (800) 826-0826 or (714) 660-8624
E-mail: uoa@deltanet.com
Home page: http://www.uoa.org

Chapter 36

Ulcers

All about Ulcers

Anatomy of an Ulcer

Ulcers in the digestive tract are like open sores. Similar to sores elsewhere, the top layer of tissue is gone, and the sore is hollowed out, like a crater. Although most ulcers heal by themselves, some do not, and get worse.

Ulcers in the stomach are called gastric ulcers. Ulcers in the duodenum, which is the first part of the small intestine just below the stomach, are called duodenal ulcers.

Causes

There have been many theories about what cause ulcers, including:

- bacterium called *Helicobacter pylori* (*H. pylori*)
- non-steroidal anti-inflammatory drugs (NSAIDs) such as aspirin, ibuprofen, or naproxen
- cigarette smoking
- excess stomach acid
- certain foods

This chapter includes text from "All about Ulcers," ©1998 TAP Pharmaceuticals, Inc, Deerfield, IL 60015, reprinted with permission; and "*H. pylori* and Peptic Ulcer," National Institute of Diabetes and Digestive and Kidney Diseases, NIH Pub. No. 97-4225, October 1997.

- emotional stress
- poor mucosal defenses
- heredity

No one reason is the cause of all ulcers. Almost all duodenal ulcers occur in people who also have *H. pylori* in their digestive tract. Some ulcers that are not due to *H. pylori* may occur in people who take non-steroidal anti-inflammatory drugs such as aspirin, ibuprofen, or naproxen, and in patients with Crohn's disease or Zollinger-Ellison syndrome.

Helicobacter Pylori. *Helicobacter pylori* (*H. pylori*) is a bacterium found in the stomachs of people with ulcers. Although many people have this organism in their stomachs, most of them don't have ulcers. On the other hand, studies show that almost everyone who has a duodenal ulcer also has *H. pylori*. Even after the ulcer has healed, most will come back within a year. But when *H. pylori* is completely eliminated from the digestive tract, the chances that a duodenal ulcer will return are greatly reduced.

Medications. Aspirin, ibuprofen, naproxen, and other medicines for pain and arthritis belong to a family of drugs called non-steroidal anti-inflammatory drugs, or NSAIDs. These drugs can increase your chances of having an ulcer because they reduce the protective layer of mucus in the stomach.

NSAID-induced ulcers can occur in people who have no evidence of *H. pylori* in their digestive tract. This suggests that there are at least two kinds of ulcer: those caused by *H. pylori* and those caused by NSAIDs. Both are aggravated by excess acid and both can be healed by acid suppression. Both types may also recur if the underlying cause is not treated.

Smoking. Smokers have more ulcers, more ulcer complications, ulcers that are more difficult to heal, and ulcers that recur more often. The reasons are not completely clear.

Excess Acid. Excess stomach acid is an important factor in the formation of ulcers. People who produce too much stomach acid are likely to develop ulcers. On the average, people who have duodenal ulcers secrete more acid than people who are ulcer-free. Healing of duodenal ulcers happens more quickly when stomach acid is reduced or eliminated by acid-suppressing drugs. Eradication of *H. pylori* may also reduce acid secretion.

Foods. There is no evidence that foods of any kind cause ulcers. All foods increase the production of stomach acid—some foods more than others—and if an ulcer already exists, the acid may cause pain. Coffee, tea, colas, and beer are all strong stimulators of stomach acid. Red and black peppers, often used in spicy foods, can injure the lining of the stomach.

Stress. Emotional and situational stresses have long been associated with ulcer flare-ups. While some studies suggest that stress does provoke ulcers, others have been unable to confirm any connection. It may be that people who are more sensitive to stress are more likely to have their ulcers aggravated by emotional problems.

Poor Mucosal Defenses. Acid that's strong enough to help digest meat and vegetables is also strong enough to cause injury to the stomach itself. To protect itself, the stomach secretes a special mucus which neutralizes the acid and covers the tissues that line the stomach. Healthy digestive tracts maintain a balance between the stomach acid and the protective mucus.

When these secretions become unbalanced, either because of too much acid or too little mucus, ulcers can develop. Other digestive juices may also play a role in ulcer formation.

Heredity. If your parents or siblings have had ulcers, the chances you will also have ulcers are greatly increased. This may be related to the transmission of *H. pylori* within families.

Symptoms

The classic symptom of duodenal ulcer is pain in the upper abdomen. The pain is usually described as "gnawing," "burning," or "cramping," and usually occurs 1-3 hours after a meal. More than half of all people with duodenal ulcers say they have abdominal pain at night.

Food may relieve ulcer pain temporarily, but because food causes acid secretion, the pain may return. Belching, bloating, or intolerance of fatty foods are common symptoms. Nausea and vomiting can also occur.

Diagnosis

If your doctor feels that the pattern of symptoms is likely due to a duodenal ulcer, he/she may want to do tests to confirm the diagnosis.

One test is an X-ray, which helps the doctor see details inside the digestive tract. Many ulcers are found this way.

Another test is called an endoscopy. It is done with a flexible tube called an endoscope, which is inserted through the mouth to view the esophagus and stomach. With an endoscope, the doctor can actually see the ulcer itself, how big it is, and if there's more than one ulcer. It can also be used to discover if something other than an ulcer is causing the problem.

Your doctor may want to test for the presence of the bacterium, *H. pylori*. This can be done during the endoscopy, with a blood test, or with a breath test.

Treatments—Lifestyle Changes

There is no evidence that diet, by itself, causes or prevents the healing of duodenal ulcers. All food causes the stomach to produce acid. You should particularly avoid any foods that aggravate your symptoms.

To minimize pain and discomfort, avoid:

- orange juice—which already has a high acid content
- alcohol—alcohol stimulates acid
- coffee or colas—it is not the caffeine, but other ingredients in these drinks that stimulate acid production
- wine, beer, and milk—all of which stimulate acid secretion

Do not smoke—nicotine inhibits healing of duodenal ulcers and may promote recurrence.

Drugs. Talk to your doctor if you take drugs like:

- aspirin
- ibuprofen
- naproxen

These drugs reduce the stomach's ability to protect itself from the harmful effects of acid.

Make sure your doctor knows about all of the drugs you are taking, whether they are prescription or over the counter.

Treatments—Medicines

Although duodenal ulcers can be healed by reducing the amount of acid in the stomach, they often will recur. One of the most exciting developments in the treatment of ulcers is the successful eradication of the bacterium *Helicobacter pylori*, because elimination of this organism from the digestive tract significantly reduces the likelihood that the ulcer will come back.

All medical treatments for the eradication of *H. pylori* involve multiple drugs, taken together. Many different combinations of acid-reducing drugs and antibiotics have been tested, and several combinations are available.

One of these combinations is a three-drug therapy that includes an acid-reducer called PREVACID®, (lansoprazole), a widely used type of penicillin called amoxicillin, and an antibiotic called BIAXIN® (clarithromycin tablets, Abbott Laboratories). Your doctor may prescribe a combination like this for your ulcer. If so, you must remember to take all of the medications as directed.

Proton Pump Inhibitors and Maintenance Therapy. Therapies that eradicate *H. pylori* have revolutionized the treatment of duodenal ulcers. By reducing the risk of ulcer recurrence, these treatments have reduced the need for long-term maintenance therapy. Some patients, however, cannot or should not take the treatments that eradicate *H. pylori*, and for them long-term maintenance therapy may be appropriate.

PREVACID belongs to a class of drugs called proton pump inhibitors. They work by shutting down the cells in the lining of the stomach that secrete stomach acid. When taken continuously over a long time, proton pump inhibitors like PREVACID can maintain the healing of duodenal ulcers for most patients. PREVACID is generally well tolerated but is not for everyone. When compared to placebo (sugar pill) the most common side effects with PREVACID include diarrhea (3.6% vs. 2.6%), abdominal pain (1.8% vs. 1.3%), and nausea (1.4% vs. 1.3%). Be sure to ask your doctor or healthcare professional if you have any questions about PREVACID.

H$_2$ Blockers. Drugs like cimetidine, ranitidine, and famotidine are histamine-receptor antagonists, or H$_2$ blockers. They also reduce the amount of acid the stomach produces. Some of these drugs have recently become available without a prescription for the treatment of heartburn and indigestion. Over-the-counter versions of these drugs should not be used for duodenal ulcers. Treatment for ulcers should be supervised by a physician.

Before proton pump inhibitors became available, H$_2$ blockers were often used continuously, at low doses, to prevent ulcer recurrence.

Within 2 to 5 years, many ulcers would recur, in spite of continued therapy.

Antacids. Although over-the-counter antacids may give temporary relief from pain, they are usually not strong enough to heal duodenal ulcers.

Summary

To heal your ulcer successfully and reduce the chances of its return, follow these simple rules:

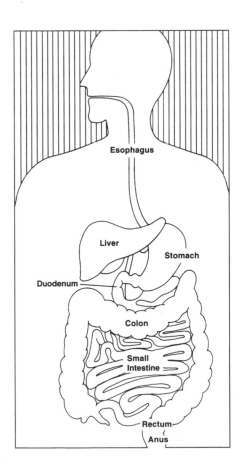

Figure 36.1. Peptic ulcers occur in the stomach or duodenum.

- Follow your doctor's advice completely.

- If that advice includes losing weight, stopping smoking, or avoiding certain foods, remember that doing so will help relieve the pain, and may help your ulcer heal faster.

- Stay in touch with your doctor and report any changes or return of symptoms.

- If your doctor prescribes any medicines, remember to take them exactly as prescribed.

By being careful, and following your doctor's recommendations, you improve the chances that your ulcer will heal and not return.

All the information about ulcer disease is not available in this chapter. For more detailed information, please see your doctor or pharmacist.

H. Pylori *and Peptic Ulcers*

What Is a Peptic Ulcer?

A peptic ulcer is a sore on the lining of the stomach or duodenum, which is the beginning of the small intestine. Peptic ulcers are common: one in every 10 Americans develops an ulcer at some time in his or her life. The main cause of peptic ulcer is bacterial infection, but some ulcers are caused by long-term use of nonsteroidal anti-inflammatory agents (NSAIDs), like aspirin and ibuprofen. In a few cases, cancerous tumors in the stomach or pancreas can cause ulcers. Peptic ulcers are not caused by spicy food or stress.

What Is H. pylori?

Helicobacter pylori (*H. pylori*) is a type of bacteria. Researchers recently discovered that *H. pylori* causes almost all peptic ulcers, accounting for 80 percent of stomach ulcers and more than 90 percent of duodenal ulcers.

H. pylori infection is common in the United States: about 20 percent of people under 40 and half of people over 60 are infected with it. Most infected people, however, do not develop ulcers. Why *H. pylori* doesn't cause ulcers in every infected person is unknown. Most likely, infection depends on characteristics of the infected person, the type of *H. pylori*, and other factors yet to be discovered.

Researchers are not certain how people become infected with *H. pylori*, but they think it may be through food or water.

Researchers have found *H. pylori* in some infected people's saliva, so the bacteria may also spread through mouth-to-mouth contact such as kissing.

How Does **H. pylori** *Cause a Peptic Ulcer?*

H. pylori weakens the protective mucous coating of the stomach and duodenum, which allows acid to get through to the sensitive lining beneath. Both the acid and the bacteria irritate the lining and cause a sore, or ulcer.

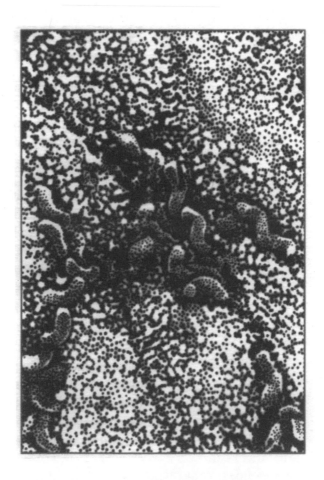

Figure 36.2. Helicobactor pylori *(*H. pylori*) bacteria.*

H. pylori is able to survive in stomach acid because it secretes enzymes that neutralize the acid. This mechanism allows *H. pylori* to make its way to the "safe" area—the protective mucous lining. Once there, the bacterium's spiral shape helps it burrow through the mucous lining.

What Are the Symptoms of an Ulcer?

Pain is the most common symptom. The pain usually:

- Is a dull, gnawing ache.
- Comes and goes for several days or weeks.
- Occurs 2 to 3 hours after a meal.
- Occurs in the middle of the night (when the stomach is empty).
- Is relieved by food.

Other symptoms include:

- Weight loss.
- Poor appetite.
- Bloating.
- Burping.
- Nausea.
- Vomiting.

Some people experience only very mild symptoms, or none at all.

Emergency Symptoms

If you have any of these symptoms, call your doctor right away:

- Sharp, sudden, persistent stomach pain.
- Bloody or black stools.
- Bloody vomit or vomit that looks like coffee grounds.

They could be signs of a serious problem, such as:

- Perforation—when the ulcer burrows through the stomach or duodenal wall.
- Bleeding—when acid or the ulcer breaks a blood vessel.
- Obstruction—when the ulcer blocks the path of food trying to leave the stomach.

How Is an H. Pylori-*Related Ulcer Diagnosed?*

Diagnosing an Ulcer. To see if symptoms are caused by an ulcer, the doctor may do an upper gastrointestinal (GI) series or an endoscopy.

An upper GI series is an x-ray of the esophagus, stomach, and duodenum. The patient drinks a chalky liquid called barium to make these organs and any ulcers show up more clearly on the x-ray.

An endoscopy is an exam with an endoscope, a thin, lighted tube with a tiny camera on the end. The patient is lightly sedated, and the doctor carefully eases the endoscope through the patient's mouth and down the throat to the stomach and duodenum. This allows the doctor to see the lining of the esophagus, stomach, and duodenum. The doctor can use the endoscope to take photos of ulcers or remove a tiny piece of tissue to view under a microscope.

Diagnosing *H. pylori*. If an ulcer is found, the doctor will test the patient for *H. pylori*. This test is important because treatment for an ulcer caused by *H. pylori* is different from that for an ulcer caused by NSAIDs.

H. pylori is diagnosed through blood, breath, and tissue tests. Blood tests are most common. They detect antibodies to *H. pylori* bacteria. Blood is taken at the doctor's office through a finger stick.

Breath tests are mainly used after treatment to see if treatment worked, but they can be used in diagnosis, too. The test is called a urea breath test.

In the doctor's office, the patient drinks a solution of urea that contains a special carbon atom. If *H. pylori* is present, it breaks down the urea, releasing the carbon. The blood carries the carbon to the lungs, where the patient exhales it. The breath test is 96 percent to 98 percent accurate.

Tissue tests are usually done using tissue removed with the endoscope. There are three types:

- The rapid urease test detects the enzyme urease, which is produced by *H. pylori*.

- A histology test allows the doctor to find and examine the actual bacteria.

- A culture test involves allowing *H. pylori* to grow in the tissue sample.

How Are **H. Pylori** *Peptic Ulcers Treated?*

H. pylori peptic ulcers are treated with drugs to kill the bacteria, to reduce stomach acid, and to protect the stomach lining. Antibiotics are used to kill the bacteria. Two types of acid-suppressing drugs might be used: H_2-blockers and proton pump inhibitors.

H_2-blockers work by blocking histamine, which stimulates acid secretion. They help reduce ulcer pain after a few weeks. Proton pump inhibitors suppress acid production by halting the mechanism that pumps the acid into the stomach. H_2-blockers and proton pump inhibitors have been prescribed alone for years as treatments for ulcers. But used alone, these drugs do not eradicate *H. pylori*, and therefore do not cure *H. pylori*-related ulcers. Bismuth subsalicylate, a component of Pepto-Bismol®, is used to protect the stomach lining from acid. It also kills *H. pylori*. Treatment usually involves a combination of antibiotics, acid suppressors, and stomach protectors.

At this time, the most proven effective treatment is a 2-week course of treatment called triple therapy. It involves taking two antibiotics to kill the bacteria and either an acid suppressor or stomach lining shield. Two-week triple therapy reduces ulcer symptoms, kills the bacteria, and prevents ulcer recurrence in more than 90 percent of patients.

Unfortunately, patients may find triple therapy complicated because it involves taking as many as 20 pills a day. Also, the antibiotics used in triple therapy may cause mild side effects such as nausea, vomiting, diarrhea, dark stools, metallic taste in the mouth, dizziness, headache, and yeast infections in women. (Most side effects can be treated with medication withdrawal.) Nevertheless, recent studies show that 2 weeks of triple therapy is ideal.

Early results of studies in other countries suggest that 1 week of triple therapy may be as effective as the 2-week therapy, with fewer side effects.

Another option is 2 weeks of dual therapy. Dual therapy involves two drugs: one antibiotic and one acid suppressor. It is not as effective as triple therapy.

Two weeks of quadruple therapy, which uses two antibiotics, an acid suppressor, and a stomach lining shield, looks promising in research studies. It is also called bismuth triple therapy.

Drugs Used to Treat H. Pylori *Peptic Ulcers*

- **Antibiotics:** metronidazole, tetracycline, clarithromycin, amoxicillin.

- **H_2-blockers:** cimetidine, ranitidine, famotidine, nizatidine.

- **Proton pump inhibitors:** omeprazole, lansoprazole.

- **Stomach-lining protector:** bismuth subsalicylate.

After Treatment. To be sure that treatment has killed all *H. pylori*, the doctor will do a followup endoscopy or breath test 6 to 12 months after treatment to check for the bacterium.

Can H. Pylori *Infection Be Prevented?*

No one knows for sure how *H. pylori* spreads, so prevention is difficult. Researchers are trying to develop a vaccine to prevent infection.

Why Don't All Doctors Automatically Check for H. Pylori?

Changing medical belief and practice takes time. For nearly 100 years, scientists and doctors thought that ulcers were caused by stress, spicy food, and alcohol. Treatment involved bed rest and a bland diet. Later, researchers added stomach acid to the list of causes and began treating ulcers with antacids.

Since *H. pylori* was discovered in 1982, studies conducted around the world have shown that using antibiotics to destroy *H. pylori* cured peptic ulcers. The National Institutes of Health released a consensus statement in 1994 confirming that *H. pylori* causes peptic ulcers. Despite the evidence, however, the medical community continues to debate *H. pylori*'s role in peptic ulcers. If you have a peptic ulcer and have not been tested for *H. pylori* infection, talk to your doctor.

Points to Remember

- A peptic ulcer is a sore in the lining of the stomach or duodenum.

- Most peptic ulcers are caused by the *H. pylori* bacterium. None are caused by spicy food or stress.

- *H. pylori* may be transmitted from person to person through contaminated food and water.

- Always wash your hands after using the bathroom and before eating.

- Antibiotics are the most effective treatment for *H. pylori* peptic ulcers.

Additional Readings

Podolski, J. L. (1996). Recent advances in peptic ulcer disease: *H. pylori* infection and its treatment. *Gastroenterology Nursing*, 19(4), 128-136.

Soll, A. H. (1996). Medical treatment of peptic ulcer disease: Practice guidelines. *Journal of the American Medical Association*, 275(8), 622-628.

National Institutes of Health, Office of the Director. (1994). NIH consensus statement: *Helicobacter pylori* in peptic ulcer disease (Vol. 12, No. 1), Bethesda, MD.

Note: The U.S. Government does not endorse or favor any specific commercial product or company. Brand names appearing in this publication are used only because they are considered essential in the context of the information.

Chapter 37

Whipple's Disease

Whipple's disease is a malabsorption disease. It interferes with the body's ability to absorb certain nutrients. The disease causes weight loss, irregular breakdown of carbohydrates and fats, resistance to insulin, and malfunctions of the immune system. When recognized and treated, Whipple's disease can be cured. Untreated, the disease is usually fatal.

Whipple's disease is caused by bacteria. It can affect any system of the body, but occurs most often in the small intestine. The disease causes lesions on the wall of the small intestine and thickening of the tissue. The villi—tiny, finger-like protrusions from the wall that help absorb nutrients—are destroyed.

Symptoms include diarrhea, intestinal bleeding, abdominal bloating and cramps, loss of appetite, weight loss, fatigue, and weakness. Arthritis and fever often occur several years before intestinal symptoms develop. Diagnosis is based on symptoms and results of a biopsy of tissue from the small intestine.

Whipple's disease is treated with antibiotics to destroy the bacteria that cause the disease. The physician may use a number of different types, doses, and schedules of antibiotics to find the best treatment. Depending on the seriousness of the disease, treatment may also include fluid and electrolyte replacement. Electrolytes are salts and other substances in body fluid that the heart and brain need to function properly. Extra iron, folate, vitamin D, calcium, and magnesium

National Digestive Diseases Information Clearinghouse, National Institute of Diabetes and Digestive and Kidney Diseases (NIDDK), March 1998.

may also be given to help compensate for the vitamins and minerals the body is not absorbing on its own.

Symptoms usually disappear after 1 to 3 months of treatment. Because relapse is common even after successful treatment, the health care team may continue to observe patients for some time.

For More Information

More information is available from:

National Organization for Rare Disorders Inc.
P.O. Box 8923
New Fairfield, CT 06812-8923
Tel: (800) 999-6673 or (203) 746-6518

Additional Information on Whipple's Disease

The National Digestive Diseases Information Clearinghouse collects resource information on digestive diseases for the Combined Health Information Database (CHID). CHID is a database produced by health-related agencies of the Federal Government. This database provides titles, abstracts, and availability information for health information and health education resources.

You may access the CHID Online website and search CHID for the most up-to-date information on Whipple's Disease.

Combined Health Information Database (CHID)
http://chid.nih.gov

Chapter 38

Zollinger-Ellison Syndrome

Zollinger-Ellison syndrome is a rare disorder that causes tumors in the pancreas and duodenum and ulcers in the stomach and duodenum. The pancreas is a gland located behind the stomach. It produces enzymes that break down fat, protein, and carbohydrates from food and hormones like insulin that break down sugar. The duodenum is the top part of the small intestine.

The tumors are cancerous in 50 percent of cases. They secrete a substance called gastrin that causes the stomach to produce too much acid, which in turn causes the stomach and duodenal ulcers (peptic ulcers). The ulcers caused by Zollinger-Ellison syndrome are more painful and less responsive to treatment than ordinary peptic ulcers. What causes people with Zollinger-Ellison syndrome to develop tumors is unknown, but the cause may be an abnormal tumor suppressor gene.

Zollinger-Ellison syndrome usually occurs in people between ages 30 and 60. Symptoms include signs of peptic ulcers: gnawing, burning pain in the abdomen; nausea; vomiting; fatigue; weakness; and weight loss. Diarrhea is also a symptom. Physicians diagnose Zollinger-Ellison syndrome through blood tests to measure levels of gastrin. They may check for ulcers by taking x-rays of the stomach and duodenum or by doing an endoscopy, which involves looking at the lining of these organs through a lighted tube.

National Digestive Diseases Information Clearinghouse, National Institute of Diabetes and Digestive and Kidney Diseases (NIDDK), March 1998.

Medications used to reduce stomach acid include cimetidine, ranitidine, famotidine, and omeprazole. Surgery to treat peptic ulcers or to remove tumors in the pancreas or duodenum are other treatment options. In serious cases, surgery to remove the entire stomach may be necessary.

For More Information

More information is available from:

National Organization for Rare Disorders Inc.
P.O. Box 8923
New Fairfield, CT 06812-8923
Tel: (800) 999-6673 or (203) 746-6518

Additional Information on Zollinger-Ellison Syndrome

The National Digestive Diseases Information Clearinghouse collects resource information on digestive diseases for the Combined Health Information Database (CHID). CHID is a database produced by health-related agencies of the Federal Government. This database provides titles, abstracts, and availability information for health information and health education resources.

You may access the CHID Online website and search CHID for the most up-to-date information on Zollinger-Ellison Syndrome.

Combined Health Information Database (CHID)
http://chid.nih.gov

Part Three

Additional Help and Information

Chapter 39

Digestive Diseases Dictionary

A

Abdomen. The area between the chest and the hips. Contains the stomach, small intestine, large intestine, liver, gallbladder, pancreas, and spleen.

Abdominal Migraine. *See* Cyclic Vomiting Syndrome.

Absorption. The way nutrients from food move from the small intestine into the cells in the body.

Accessory Digestive Organs. Organs that help with digestion but are not part of the digestive tract. These organs are the tongue, glands in the mouth that make saliva, pancreas, liver, and gallbladder.

Achalasia. A rare disorder of the esophagus. The muscle at the end of the esophagus does not relax enough for the passage to open properly.

Achlorhydria. A lack of hydrochloric acid in stomach juice.

Activated Charcoal. An over-the-counter product that may help relieve intestinal gas.

National Digestive Diseases Information Clearinghouse, National Institute of Diabetes and Digestive and Kidney Diseases (NIDDK), NIH Pub. No. 97-2750, March 1997.

Acute. A disorder that is sudden and severe but lasts only a short time.

Aerophagia. A condition that occurs when a person swallows too much air. Causes gas and frequent belching.

Alactasia. An inherited condition causing the lack of the enzyme needed to digest milk sugar.

Alagille Syndrome. A condition of babies in their first year. The bile ducts in the liver disappear, and the bile ducts outside the liver get very narrow. May lead to a buildup of bile in the liver and damage to liver cells and other organs.

Alimentary Canal. *See* Gastrointestinal (GI) Tract.

Allergy. A condition in which the body is not able to tolerate certain foods, animals, plants, or other substances.

Amebiasis. An acute or chronic infection. Symptoms vary from mild diarrhea to frequent watery diarrhea and loss of water and fluids in the body. *See also* Gastroenteritis.

Amino Acids. The basic building blocks of proteins. The body makes many amino acids. Others come from food and the body breaks them down for use by cells. *See also* Protein.

Anal Fissure. A small tear in the anus that may cause itching, pain, or bleeding.

Anal Fistula. A channel that develops between the anus and the skin. Most fistulas are the result of an abscess (infection) that spreads to the skin.

Anastomosis. An operation to connect two body parts. An example is an operation in which a part of the colon is removed and the two remaining ends are rejoined.

Anemia. Not enough red blood, red blood cells, or hemoglobin in the body. Hemoglobin is a protein in the blood that contains iron.

Angiodysplasia. Abnormal or enlarged blood vessels in the gastrointestinal tract.

Angiography. An x-ray that uses dye to detect bleeding in the gastrointestinal tract.

Anorectal Atresia. Lack of a normal opening between the rectum and anus.

Anoscopy. A test to look for fissures, fistulae, and hemorrhoids. The doctor uses a special instrument, called an anoscope, to look into the anus.

Antacids. Medicines that balance acids and gas in the stomach. Examples are Maalox®, Mylanta®, and Di-Gel®.

Anticholinergics. Medicines that calm muscle spasms in the intestine. Examples are dicyclomine (Bentyl®) and hyoscyamine (Levsin®).

Antidiarrheals. Medicines that help control diarrhea. An example is loperamide (Imodium®).

Antiemetics. Medicines that prevent and control nausea and vomiting. Examples are promethazine (Phenergan®) and prochlorperazine (Compazine®).

Antispasmodics. Medicines that help reduce or stop muscle spasms in the intestines. Examples are dicyclomine (Bentyl®) and atropine (Donnatal®).

Antrectomy. An operation to remove the upper portion of the stomach, called the antrum. This operation helps reduce the amount of stomach acid. It is used when a person has complications from ulcers.

Anus. The opening at the end of the digestive tract where bowel contents leave the body.

Appendectomy. An operation to remove the appendix.

Appendicitis. Reddening, irritation (inflammation), and pain in the appendix caused by infection, scarring, or blockage.

Appendix. A 4-inch pouch attached to the first part of the large intestine (cecum). No one knows what function the appendix has, if any.

Ascending Colon. The part of the colon on the right side of the abdomen.

Ascites. A buildup of fluid in the abdomen. Ascites is usually caused by severe liver disease such as cirrhosis.

Asymptomatic. The condition of having a disease, but without any symptoms of it.

Atonic Colon. Lack of normal muscle tone or strength in the colon. This is caused by the overuse of laxatives or by Hirschsprung's disease. It may result in chronic constipation. Also called lazy colon. *See* Hirschsprung's Disease.

Atresia. Lack of a normal opening from the esophagus, intestines, or anus.

Atrophic Gastritis. Chronic irritation of the stomach lining. Causes the stomach lining and glands to wither away.

Autoimmune Hepatitis. A liver disease caused when the body's immune system destroys liver cells for no known reason.

B

Barium. A chalky liquid used to coat the inside of organs so that they will show up on an x-ray.

Barium Enema X-Ray. *See* Lower GI Series.

Barium Meal. *See* Upper GI Series.

Barrett's Esophagus. Peptic ulcer of the lower esophagus. It is caused by the presence of cells that normally stay in the stomach lining.

Belching. Noisy release of gas from the stomach through the mouth. Also called burping.

Bernstein Test. A test to find out if heartburn is caused by acid in the esophagus. The test involves dripping a mild acid, similar to stomach acid, through a tube placed in the esophagus.

Bezoar. A ball of food, mucus, vegetable fiber, hair, or other material that cannot be digested in the stomach. Bezoars can cause blockage, ulcers, and bleeding.

Bile. Fluid made by the liver and stored in the gallbladder. Bile helps break down fats and gets rid of wastes in the body.

Bile Acids. Acids made by the liver that work with bile to break down fats.

Bile Ducts. Tubes that carry bile from the liver to the gallbladder for storage and to the small intestine for use in digestion.

Biliary Atresia. A condition present from birth in which the bile ducts inside or outside the liver do not have normal openings. Bile becomes trapped in the liver, causing jaundice and cirrhosis. Without surgery the condition may cause death.

Biliary Dyskinesia. *See* Postcholecystectomy Syndrome.

Biliary Stricture. A narrowing of the biliary tract from scar tissue. The scar tissue may result from injury, disease, pancreatitis, infection, or gallstones. *See also* Stricture.

Biliary System. *See* Biliary Tract.

Biliary Tract. The gallbladder and the bile ducts. Also called biliary system or biliary tree.

Biliary Tree. *See* Biliary Tract.

Bilirubin. The substance formed when hemoglobin breaks down. Bilirubin gives bile its color. Bilirubin is normally passed in stool. Too much bilirubin causes jaundice.

Bismuth Subsalicylate. A nonprescription medicine such as Pepto-Bismol®. Used to treat diarrhea, heartburn, indigestion, and nausea. It is also part of the treatment for ulcers caused by the bacterium *Helicobacter pylori*.

Bloating. Fullness or swelling in the abdomen that often occurs after meals.

Borborygmi. Rumbling sounds caused by gas moving through the intestines (stomach "growling").

Bowel. Another word for the small and large intestines.

Bowel Movement. Body wastes passed through the rectum and anus.

Bowel Prep. The process used to clean the colon with enemas and a special drink. Used before surgery of the colon, colonoscopy, or barium x-ray. *See also* Lavage.

Budd-Chiari Syndrome. A rare liver disease in which the veins that drain blood from the liver are blocked or narrowed.

Bulking Agents. Laxatives that make bowel movements soft and easy to pass.

Burping. *See* Belching.

C

Calculi. Stones or solid lumps such as gallstones.

Campylobacter pylori. The original name for the bacterium that causes ulcers. The new name is *Helicobacter pylori*. *See also Helicobacter pylori*.

Candidiasis. A mild infection caused by the *Candida* fungus, which lives naturally in the gastrointestinal tract. Infection occurs when a change in the body, such as surgery, causes the fungus to overgrow suddenly.

Carbohydrates. One of the three main classes of food and a source of energy. Carbohydrates are the sugars and starches found in breads, cereals, fruits, and vegetables. During digestion, carbohydrates are changed into a simple sugar called glucose. Glucose is stored in the liver until cells need it for energy.

Caroli's Disease. An inherited condition. Bile ducts in the liver are enlarged and may cause irritation, infection, or gallstones.

Cathartics. *See* Laxatives.

Catheter. A thin, flexible tube that carries fluids into or out of the body.

Cecostomy. A tube that goes through the skin into the beginning of the large intestine to remove gas or feces. This is a short-term way to protect part of the colon while it heals after surgery.

Cecum. The beginning of the large intestine. The cecum is connected to the lower part of the small intestine, called the ileum.

Celiac Disease. Inability to digest and absorb gliadin, the protein found in wheat. Undigested gliadin causes damage to the lining of the small intestine. This prevents absorption of nutrients from other foods. Celiac disease is also called celiac sprue, gluten intolerance, and nontropical sprue.

Celiac Sprue. *See* Celiac Disease.

Chlorhydria. Too much hydrochloric acid in the stomach.

Cholangiography. A series of x-rays of the bile ducts.

Cholangitis. Irritated or infected bile ducts.

Cholecystectomy. An operation to remove the gallbladder.

Cholecystitis. An irritated gallbladder.

Cholecystogram, Oral. An x-ray of the gallbladder and bile ducts. The patient takes pills containing a special dye to make the organs show up in the x-ray. Also called oral cholecystography.

Cholecystography, Oral. *See* Cholecystogram, Oral.

Cholecystokinin. A hormone released in the small intestine. Causes muscles in the gallbladder and the colon to tighten and relax.

Choledocholithiasis. Gallstones in the bile ducts.

Cholelithiasis. Gallstones in the gallbladder.

Cholestasis. Blocked bile ducts. Often caused by gallstones.

Cholesterol. A fat-like substance in the body. The body makes and needs some cholesterol, which also comes from foods such as butter and egg yolks. Too much cholesterol may cause gallstones. It also may cause fat to build up in the arteries. This may cause a disease that slows or stops blood flow.

Chronic. A term that refers to disorders that last a long time, often years.

251

Chyme. A thick liquid made of partially digested food and stomach juices. This liquid is made in the stomach and moves into the small intestine for further digestion.

Cirrhosis. A chronic liver condition caused by scar tissue and cell damage. Cirrhosis makes it hard for the liver to remove poisons (toxins) like alcohol and drugs from the blood. These toxins build up in the blood and may affect brain function.

***Clostridium difficile* (*C. difficile*).** Bacteria naturally present in the large intestine. These bacteria make a substance that can cause a serious infection called pseudomembranous colitis in people taking antibiotics.

Colectomy. An operation to remove all or part of the colon.

Colic. Attacks of abdominal pain, caused by muscle spasms in the intestines. Colic is common in infants.

Colitis. Irritation of the colon.

Collagenous Colitis. A type of colitis. Caused by an abnormal band of collagen, a thread-like protein.

Colon. *See* Large Intestine.

Colonic Inertia. A condition of the colon. Colon muscles do not work properly, causing constipation.

Colonoscopy. A test to look into the rectum and colon. The doctor uses a long, flexible, narrow tube with a light and tiny lens on the end. This tube is called a colonoscope.

Colonoscopic Polypectomy. The removal of tumor-like growths (polyps) using a device inserted through a colonoscope.

Colon Polyps. Small, fleshy, mushroom-shaped growths in the colon.

Coloproctectomy. *See* Proctocolectomy.

Colorectal Cancer. Cancer that occurs in the colon (large intestine) or the rectum (the end of the large intestine). A number of digestive diseases may increase a person's risk of colorectal cancer, including polyposis and Zollinger-Ellison Syndrome.

Colorectal Transit Study. A test to see how food moves through the colon. The patient swallows capsules that contain small markers. An x-ray tracks the movement of the capsules through the colon.

Colostomy. An operation that makes it possible for stool to leave the body after the rectum has been removed. The surgeon makes an opening in the abdomen and attaches the colon to it. A temporary colostomy may be done to let the rectum heal from injury or other surgery.

Common Bile Duct. The tube that carries bile from the liver to the small intestine.

Common Bile Duct Obstruction. A blockage of the common bile duct, often caused by gallstones.

Computed Tomography (CT) Scan. An x-ray that produces three-dimensional pictures of the body. Also known as computed axial tomography (CAT) scan.

Constipation. A condition in which the stool becomes hard and dry. A person who is constipated usually has fewer than three bowel movements in a week. Bowel movements may be painful.

Continence. The ability to hold in a bowel movement or urine.

Continent Ileostomy. An operation to create a pouch from part of the small intestine. Stool that collects in the pouch is removed by inserting a small tube through an opening made in the abdomen. *See also* Ileostomy.

Corticosteroids. Medicines such as cortisone and hydrocortisone. These medicines reduce irritation from Crohn's disease and ulcerative colitis. They may be taken either by mouth or as suppositories.

Crohn's Disease. A chronic form of inflammatory bowel disease. Crohn's disease causes severe irritation in the gastrointestinal tract. It usually affects the lower small intestine (called the ileum) or the colon, but it can affect the entire gastrointestinal tract. Also called regional enteritis and ileitis. *See also* Inflammatory Bowel Disease (IBD) and Granuloma.

Cryptosporidia. A parasite that can cause gastrointestinal infection and diarrhea. *See also* Gastroenteritis.

Cyclic Vomiting Syndrome (CVS). Sudden, repeated attacks of severe vomiting (especially in children), nausea, and physical exhaustion with no apparent cause. Can last from a few hours to 10 days. The episodes begin and end suddenly. Loss of fluids in the body and changes in chemicals in the body can require immediate medical attention. Also called abdominal migraine.

Cystic Duct. The tube that carries bile from the gallbladder into the common bile duct and the small intestine.

Cystic Duct Obstruction. A blockage of the cystic duct, often caused by gallstones.

D

Defecation. The passage of bowel contents through the rectum and anus.

Defecography. An x-ray of the anus and rectum to see how the muscles work to move stool. The patient sits on a toilet placed inside the x-ray machine.

Dehydration. Loss of fluids from the body, often caused by diarrhea. May result in loss of important salts and minerals.

Delayed Gastric Emptying. *See* Gastroparesis.

Dermatitis Herpetiformis. A skin disorder associated with celiac disease. *See also* Celiac Disease.

Descending Colon. The part of the colon where stool is stored. Located on the left side of the abdomen.

Diaphragm. The muscle wall between the chest and the abdomen. It is the major muscle that the body uses for breathing.

Diarrhea. Frequent, loose, and watery bowel movements. Common causes include gastrointestinal infections, irritable bowel syndrome, medicines, and malabsorption.

Dietitian. An expert in nutrition who helps people plan what and how much food to eat.

Digestants. Medicines that aid or stimulate digestion. An example is a digestive enzyme such as Lactaid® for people with lactase deficiency.

Digestion. The process the body uses to break down food into simple substances for energy, growth, and cell repair.

Digestive System. The organs in the body that break down and absorb food. Organs that make up the digestive system are the mouth, esophagus, stomach, small intestine, large intestine, rectum, and anus. Organs that help with digestion but are not part of the digestive tract are the tongue, glands in the mouth that make saliva, pancreas, liver, and gallbladder.

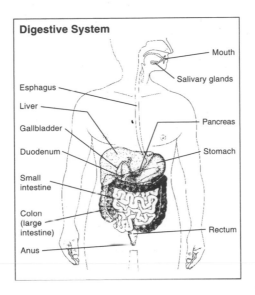

Figure 39.1. *The organs of the digestive system and accessory digestive organs.*

Digestive Tract. *See* Gastrointestinal (GI) Tract.

Distention. Bloating or swelling of the abdomen.

Diverticula. Plural form of diverticulum. *See* Diverticulum.

Diverticulitis. A condition that occurs when small pouches in the colon (diverticula) become infected or irritated. Also called left-sided appendicitis.

Diverticulosis. A condition that occurs when small pouches (diverticula) push outward through weak spots in the colon.

Diverticulum. A small pouch in the colon. These pouches are not painful or harmful unless they become infected or irritated.

Dry Mouth. *See* Xerostomia.

Dubin-Johnson Syndrome. An inherited form of chronic jaundice (yellow tint to the skin and eyes) that has no known cause.

Dumping Syndrome. A condition that occurs when food moves too fast from the stomach into the small intestine. Symptoms are nausea, pain, weakness, and sweating. This syndrome most often affects people who have had stomach operations. Also called rapid gastric emptying.

Duodenal Ulcer. An ulcer in the lining of the first part of the small intestine (duodenum).

Duodenitis. An irritation of the first part of the small intestine (duodenum).

Duodenum. The first part of the small intestine.

Dysentery. An infectious disease of the colon. Symptoms include bloody, mucus-filled diarrhea; abdominal pain; fever; and loss of fluids from the body.

Dyspepsia. *See* Indigestion.

Dysphagia. Problems in swallowing food or liquid, usually caused by blockage or injury to the esophagus.

E

Eagle-Barrett Syndrome. *See* Prune Belly Syndrome.

Electrocoagulation. A procedure that uses an electrical current passed through an endoscope to stop bleeding in the digestive tract and to remove affected tissue.

Electrolytes. Chemicals such as salts and minerals needed for various functions in the body.

Encopresis. Accidental passage of a bowel movement. A common disorder in children.

Endoscope. A small, flexible tube with a light and a lens on the end. It is used to look into the esophagus, stomach, duodenum, colon, or rectum. It can also be used to take tissue from the body for testing or to take color photographs of the inside of the body. Colonoscopes and sigmoidoscopes are types of endoscopes.

Endoscopic Papillotomy. *See* Endoscopic Sphincterotomy.

Endoscopic Retrograde Cholangiopancreatography (ERCP). A test using an x-ray to look into the bile and pancreatic ducts. The doctor inserts an endoscope through the mouth into the duodenum and bile ducts. Dye is sent through the tube into the ducts. The dye makes the ducts show up on an x-ray.

Endoscopic Sphincterotomy. An operation to cut the muscle between the common bile duct and the pancreatic duct. The operation uses a catheter and a wire to remove gallstones or other blockages. Also called endoscopic papillotomy.

Endoscopy. A procedure that uses an endoscope to diagnose or treat a condition.

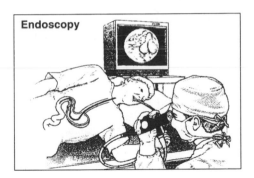

Figure 39.2. Endoscopy is used to diagnose or treat problems in the esophagus, stomach, and duodenum.

Enema. A liquid put into the rectum to clear out the bowel or to administer drugs or food.

Enteral Nutrition. A way to provide food through a tube placed in the nose, the stomach, or the small intestine. A tube in the nose is called a nasogastric or nasoenteral tube. A tube that goes through the skin into the stomach is called a gastrostomy or percutaneous endoscopic gastrostomy (PEG). A tube into the small intestine is called a jejunostomy or percutaneous endoscopic jejunostomy (PEJ) tube. Also called tube feeding. *See also* Gastrostomy and Jejunostomy.

Enteritis. An irritation of the small intestine.

Enterocele. A hernia in the intestine. *See* also Hernia.

Enteroscopy. An examination of the small intestine with an endoscope. The endoscope is inserted through the mouth and stomach into the small intestine.

Enterostomal Therapy (ET) Nurse. A nurse who cares for patients with an ostomy. *See also* Ostomy.

Enterostomy. An ostomy, or opening, into the intestine through the abdominal wall.

Enzyme-Linked Immunosorbent Assay (ELISA). A blood test used to find *Helicobacter pylori* bacteria. Also used to diagnose an ulcer.

Eosinophilic Gastroenteritis. Infection and swelling of the lining of the stomach, small intestine, or large intestine. The infection is caused by white blood cells (eosinophils).

Epithelial Cells. One of many kinds of cells that form the epithelium and absorb nutrients. *See also* Epithelium.

Epithelium. The inner and outer tissue covering digestive tract organs.

ERCP. *See* Endoscopic Retrograde Cholangiopancreatography (ERCP).

Eructation. Belching.

Erythema Nodosum. Red swellings or sores on the lower legs during flare-ups of Crohn's disease and ulcerative colitis. These sores show that the disease is active. They usually go away when the disease is treated.

Escherichia coli. Bacteria that cause infection and irritation of the large intestine. The bacteria are spread by unclean water, dirty cooking utensils, or undercooked meat. *See also* Gastroenteritis.

Esophageal Atresia. A birth defect. The esophagus lacks the opening to allow food to pass into the stomach.

Esophageal Manometry. A test to measure muscle tone in the esophagus.

Esophageal pH Monitoring. A test to measure the amount of acid in the esophagus.

Esophageal Reflux. *See* Gastroesophageal Reflux Disease.

Esophageal Spasms. Muscle cramps in the esophagus that cause pain in the chest.

Esophageal Stricture. A narrowing of the esophagus often caused by acid flowing back from the stomach. This condition may require surgery.

Esophageal Ulcer. A sore in the esophagus. Caused by long-term inflammation or damage from the residue of pills. The ulcer may cause chest pain.

Esophageal Varices. Stretched veins in the esophagus that occur when the liver is not working properly. If the veins burst, the bleeding can cause death.

Esophagitis. An irritation of the esophagus, usually caused by acid that flows up from the stomach.

Esophagogastroduodenoscopy (EGD). Exam of the upper digestive tract using an endoscope. *See* Endoscopy.

Esophagus. The organ that connects the mouth to the stomach. Also called gullet.

Excrete. To get rid of waste from the body.

Extrahepatic Biliary Tree. The bile ducts located outside the liver.

F

Failure to Thrive. A condition that occurs when a baby does not grow normally.

Familial Polyposis. An inherited disease causing many polyps in the colon. The polyps often cause cancer.

Fats. One of the three main classes of food and a source of energy in the body. Bile dissolves fats, and enzymes break them down. This process moves fats into cells.

Fatty Liver. The buildup of fat in liver cells. The most common cause is alcoholism. Other causes include obesity, diabetes, and pregnancy. Also called steatosis.

Fecal Fat Test. A test to measure the body's ability to break down and absorb fat. The patient eats a fat-free diet for 2 to 3 days before the test and collects stool samples for examination.

Fecal Incontinence. Being unable to hold stool in the colon and rectum.

Fecal Occult Blood Test (FOBT). A test to see whether there is blood in the stool that is not visible to the naked eye. A sample of stool is placed on a chemical strip that will change color if blood is present. Hidden blood in the stool is a common symptom of colorectal cancer.

Feces. Stool.

Fermentation. The process of bacteria breaking down undigested food and releasing alcohols, acids, and gases.

Fiber. A substance in foods that comes from plants. Fiber helps with digestion by keeping stool soft so that it moves smoothly through the colon. Soluble fiber dissolves in water. Soluble fiber is found in beans, fruit, and oat products. Insoluble fiber does not dissolve in water. Insoluble fiber is found in whole-grain products and vegetables.

Fistula. An abnormal passage between two organs or between an organ and the outside of the body. Caused when damaged tissues come into contact with each other and join together while healing.

Flatulence. Excessive gas in the stomach or intestine. May cause bloating.

Flatus. Gas passed through the rectum.

Foodborne Illness. An acute gastrointestinal infection caused by food that contains harmful bacteria. Symptoms include diarrhea, abdominal pain, fever, and chills. Also called food poisoning.

Fulminant Hepatic Failure (FHF). Liver failure that occurs suddenly in a previously healthy person. The most common causes of FHF are acute hepatitis, acetaminophen overdose, and liver damage from prescription drugs.

Functional Disorders. Disorders such as irritable bowel syndrome. These conditions result from poor nerve and muscle function. Symptoms such as gas, pain, constipation, and diarrhea come back again and again, but there are no signs of disease or damage. Emotional stress can trigger symptoms. Also called motility disorders.

Fungus. A mold or yeast such as *Candidiasis* that may cause infection.

G

Galactose. A type of sugar in milk products and sugar beets. The body also makes galactose.

Galactosemia. Buildup of galactose in the blood. Caused by lack of one of the enzymes needed to break down galactose into glucose.

Gallbladder. The organ that stores the bile made in the liver. Connected to the liver by bile ducts. The gallbladder can store about 1 cup of bile. Eating signals the gallbladder to empty the bile through the bile ducts to help digest fats.

Gallstones. The solid masses or stones made of cholesterol or bilirubin that form in the gallbladder or bile ducts.

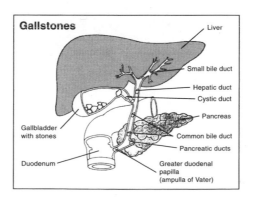

Figure 39.3. *Gallstones, solid masses made of cholesterol or bilirubin, form in the gallbladder or bile ducts.*

Gardner's Syndrome. A condition in which many polyps form throughout the digestive tract. Because these polyps are likely to cause cancer, the colon and rectum are often removed to prevent colorectal cancer.

Gas. Air that comes from normal breakdown of food. The gases are passed out of the body through the rectum (flatus) or the mouth (burp).

Gastrectomy. An operation to remove all or part of the stomach.

Gastric. Related to the stomach.

Gastric Juices. Liquids produced in the stomach to help break down food and kill bacteria.

Gastric Resection. An operation to remove part or all of the stomach.

Gastric Ulcer. *See* Stomach Ulcer.

Gastrin. A hormone released after eating. Gastrin causes the stomach to produce more acid.

Gastritis. An inflammation of the stomach lining.

Gastrocolic Reflex. Increase of muscle movement in the gastrointestinal tract when food enters an empty stomach. May cause the urge to have a bowel movement right after eating.

Gastroenteritis. An infection or irritation of the stomach and intestines. May be caused by bacteria or parasites from spoiled food or unclean water. Other causes include eating food that irritates the stomach lining and emotional upsets such as anger, fear, or stress. Symptoms include diarrhea, nausea, vomiting, and abdominal cramping. *See also* Infectious Diarrhea and Travelers' Diarrhea.

Gastroenterologist. A doctor who specializes in digestive diseases.

Gastroenterology. The field of medicine concerned with the function and disorders of the digestive system.

Gastroesophageal Reflux Disease (GERD). Flow of the stomach's contents back up into the esophagus. Happens when the muscle between the esophagus and the stomach (the lower esophageal sphincter) is weak or relaxes when it shouldn't. May cause esophagitis. Also called esophageal reflux or reflux esophagitis.

Gastrointestinal (GI). Related to the gastrointestinal tract.

Gastrointestinal (GI) Tract. The large, muscular tube that extends from the mouth to the anus, where the movement of muscles and release of hormones and enzymes digest food. Also called the alimentary canal or digestive tract.

Gastroparesis. Nerve or muscle damage in the stomach. Causes slow digestion and emptying, vomiting, nausea, or bloating. Also called delayed gastric emptying.

Gastrostomy. An artificial opening from the stomach to a hole (stoma) in the abdomen where a feeding tube is inserted. *See also* Enteral Nutrition.

GERD. *See* Gastroesophageal Reflux Disease.

GI. *See* Gastrointestinal.

Giant Hypertrophic Gastritis. *See* Ménétrier's Disease.

Giardiasis. An infection with the parasite *Giardia lamblia* from spoiled food or unclean water. May cause diarrhea. *See also* Gastroenteritis.

Gilbert Syndrome. A buildup of bilirubin in the blood. Caused by lack of a liver enzyme needed to break down bilirubin. *See also* Bilirubin.

Globus Sensation. A constant feeling of a lump in the throat. Usually related to stress.

Glucose. A simple sugar the body manufactures from carbohydrates in the diet. Glucose is the body's main source of energy. *See also* Carbohydrates.

Gluten. A protein found in wheat, rye, barley, and oats. In people who can't digest it, gluten damages the lining of the small intestine or causes sores on the skin.

Gluten Intolerance. *See* Celiac Disease.

Gluten Sensitive Enteropathy. A general term that refers to celiac disease and dermatitis herpetiformis.

Glycogen. A sugar stored in the liver and muscles. It releases glucose into the blood when cells need it for energy. Glycogen is the chief source of stored fuel in the body.

Glycogen Storage Diseases. A group of birth defects. These diseases change the way the liver breaks down glycogen. *See also* Glycogen.

Granuloma. A mass of red, irritated tissue in the GI tract found in Crohn's disease.

Granulomatous Colitis. Another name for Crohn's disease of the colon.

Granulomatous Enteritis. Another name for Crohn's disease of the small intestine.

Gullet. *See* Esophagus.

Gut. *See* Intestines.

H

H$_2$-Blockers. Medicines that reduce the amount of acid the stomach produces. They block histamine$_2$. Histamine signals the stomach to make acid. Prescription H$_2$-blockers are cimetidine (Tagamet®), famotidine (Pepcid®), nizatidine (Axid®), and ranitidine (Zantac®). They are used to treat ulcer symptoms. Nonprescription H$_2$-blockers are Zantac 75®, Axid AR®, Pepcid-AC®, and Tagamet-HB®. They are for GERD, heartburn, and acid indigestion.

Heartburn. A painful, burning feeling in the chest. Heartburn is caused by stomach acid flowing back into the esophagus. Changing the diet and other habits can help to prevent heartburn. Heartburn may be a symptom of GERD. *See also* Gastroesophageal Reflux Disease (GERD).

Helicobacter pylori (H. pylori). A spiral-shaped bacterium found in the stomach. *H. pylori* damages stomach and duodenal tissue, causing ulcers. Previously called *Campylobacter pylori*.

Hemochromatosis. A disease that occurs when the body absorbs too much iron. The body stores the excess iron in the liver, pancreas, and other organs. May cause cirrhosis of the liver. Also called iron overload disease.

Hemorrhoidectomy. An operation to remove hemorrhoids.

Hemorrhoids. Swollen blood vessels in and around the anus and lower rectum. Continual straining to have a bowel movement causes them to stretch and swell. They cause itching, pain, and sometimes bleeding.

Hepatic. Related to the liver.

Hepatic Coma. *See* Hepatic Encephalopathy.

Hepatic Encephalopathy. A condition that may cause loss of consciousness and coma. It is usually the result of advanced liver disease. Also called hepatic coma.

Hepatitis. Irritation of the liver that sometimes causes permanent damage. Hepatitis may be caused by viruses or by medicines or alcohol. Hepatitis has the following forms:

- *Hepatitis A:* A virus most often spread by unclean food and water.

- *Hepatitis B:* A virus commonly spread by sexual intercourse or blood transfusion, or from mother to newborn at birth. Another way it spreads is by using a needle that was used by an infected person. Hepatitis B is more common and much more easily spread than the AIDS virus and may lead to cirrhosis and liver cancer.

- *Hepatitis C:* A virus spread by blood transfusion and possibly by sexual intercourse or sharing needles with infected people. Hepatitis C may lead to cirrhosis and liver cancer. Hepatitis C used to be called non-A, non-B hepatitis.

- *Hepatitis D (Delta):* A virus that occurs mostly in people who take illegal drugs by using needles. Only people who have hepatitis B can get hepatitis D.

- *Hepatitis E:* A virus spread mostly through unclean water. This type of hepatitis is common in developing countries. It has not occurred in the United States.

Hepatitis B Immunoglobulin (HBIg). A shot that gives short-term protection from the hepatitis B virus.

Hepatitis B Vaccine. A shot to prevent hepatitis B. The vaccine tells the body to make its own protection (antibodies) against the virus.

Hepatologist. A doctor who specializes in liver diseases.

Hepatology. The field of medicine concerned with the functions and disorders of the liver.

Hepatotoxicity. How much damage a medicine or other substance does to the liver.

Hernia. The part of an internal organ that pushes through an opening in the organ's wall. Most hernias occur in the abdominal area.

Herniorrhaphy. An operation to repair a hernia.

Hiatal Hernia (Hiatus Hernia). A small opening in the diaphragm that allows the upper part of the stomach to move up into the chest. Causes heartburn from stomach acid flowing back up through the opening. *See also* Diaphragm.

Hirschsprung's Disease. A birth defect in which some nerve cells are lacking in the large intestine. The intestine cannot move stool through, so the intestine gets blocked. Causes the abdomen to swell. *See also* Megacolon.

Hormone. A substance in the body that regulates certain organs. Hormones such as gastrin help in breaking down food. Some hormones come from cells in the stomach and small intestine.

Hydrochloric Acid. An acid made in the stomach. Hydrochloric acid works with pepsin and other enzymes to break down proteins.

Hydrogen Breath Test. A test for lactose intolerance. It measures breath samples for too much hydrogen. The body makes too much hydrogen when lactose is not broken down properly in the small intestine.

Hyperalimentation. *See* Parenteral Nutrition.

Hyperbilirubinemia. Too much bilirubin in the blood. Symptoms include jaundice. This condition occurs when the liver does not work normally. *See also* Jaundice.

I

IBD. *See* Inflammatory Bowel Disease (IBD).

IBS. *See* Irritable Bowel Syndrome (IBS).

Ileal. Related to the ileum, the lowest end of the small intestine.

Ileal Pouch. *See* Ileoanal Reservoir.

Ileitis. *See* Crohn's Disease.

Ileoanal Anastomosis. *See* Ileoanal Pull-Through.

Ileoanal Pull-Through. An operation to remove the colon and inner lining of the rectum. The outer muscle of the rectum is not touched. The bottom end of the small intestine (ileum) is pulled through the remaining rectum and joined to the anus. Stool can be passed normally. Also called ileoanal anastomosis.

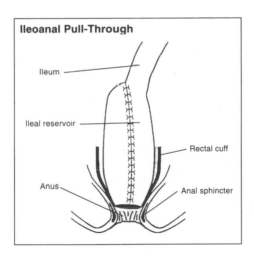

Ileoanal Pull-Through

Ileum

Ileal reservoir

Rectal cuff

Anus

Anal sphincter

Figure 39.4. The bottom end of the small intestine, called the ileum, is joined to the anus.

Ileoanal Reservoir. An operation to remove the colon, upper rectum, and part of the lower rectum. An internal pouch is created from the remaining intestine to hold stool. The operation may be done in two stages. The pouch may also be called a J-pouch or W-pouch.

Ileocecal Valve. A valve that connects the lower part of the small intestine and the upper part of the large intestine (ileum and cecum). Controls the flow of fluid in the intestines and prevents backflow.

Ileocolitis. Irritation of the lower part of the small intestine (ileum) and colon.

Ileostomy. An operation that makes it possible for stool to leave the body after the colon and rectum are removed. The surgeon makes an opening in the abdomen and attaches the bottom of the small intestine (ileum) to it.

Ileum. The lower end of the small intestine.

Impaction. The trapping of an object in a body passage. Examples are stones in the bile duct or hardened stool in the colon.

Imperforate Anus. A birth defect in which the anal canal fails to develop. The condition is treated with an operation.

Indigestion. Poor digestion. Symptoms include heartburn, nausea, bloating, and gas. Also called dyspepsia.

Infectious Diarrhea. Diarrhea caused by infection from bacteria, viruses, or parasites. *See also* Travelers' Diarrhea and Gastroenteritis.

Infectious Gastroenteritis. *See* Gastroenteritis.

Inflammatory Bowel Disease (IBD). Long-lasting problems that cause irritation and ulcers in the GI tract. The most common disorders are ulcerative colitis and Crohn's disease.

Inguinal Hernia. A small part of the large or small intestine or bladder that pushes into the groin. May cause pain and feelings of pressure or burning in the groin. Often requires surgery.

Intestines. *See* Large Intestine and Small Intestine. Also called gut.

Intestinal Flora. The bacteria, yeasts, and fungi that grow normally in the intestines.

Intestinal Mucosa. The surface lining of the intestines where the cells absorb nutrients.

Intestinal Pseudo-Obstruction. A disorder that causes symptoms of blockage, but no actual blockage. Causes constipation, vomiting, and pain. *See also* Obstruction.

Intussusception. A rare disorder. A part of the intestines folds into another part of the intestines, causing blockage. Most common in infants. Can be treated with an operation.

Iron Overload Disease. *See* Hemochromatosis.

Irritable Bowel Syndrome (IBS). A disorder that comes and goes. Nerves that control the muscles in the GI tract are too active. The GI tract becomes sensitive to food, stool, gas, and stress. Causes abdominal pain, bloating, and constipation or diarrhea. Also called spastic colon or mucous colitis.

Ischemic Colitis. Decreased blood flow to the colon. Causes fever, pain, and bloody diarrhea.

J

Jaundice. A symptom of many disorders. Jaundice causes the skin and eyes to turn yellow from too much bilirubin in the blood. *See also* Hyperbilirubinemia.

Jejunum. The middle section of the small intestine between the duodenum and ileum.

Jejunostomy. An operation to create an opening of the jejunum to a hole (stoma) in the abdomen. *See also* Enteral Nutrition.

K

Kupffer's Cells. Cells that line the liver. These cells remove waste such as bacteria from the blood.

L

Lactase. An enzyme in the small intestine needed to digest milk sugar (lactose).

Lactase Deficiency. Lack of the lactase enzyme. Causes lactose intolerance.

Lactose. The sugar found in milk. The body breaks lactose down into galactose and glucose.

Lactose Intolerance. Being unable to digest lactose, the sugar in milk. This condition occurs because the body does not produce the lactase enzyme.

Lactose Tolerance Test. A test for lactase deficiency. The patient drinks a liquid that contains milk sugar. Then the patient's blood is tested; the test measures the amount of milk sugar in the blood.

Laparoscope. A thin tube with a tiny video camera attached. Used to look inside the body and see the surface of organs. *See also* Endoscope.

Laparoscopic Cholecystectomy. An operation to remove the gallbladder. The doctor inserts a laparoscope (*See* Laparoscope) and other surgical instruments through small holes in the abdomen. The camera allows the doctor to see the gallbladder on a television screen. The doctor removes the gallbladder through the holes.

Laparoscopy. A test that uses a laparoscope to look at and take tissue from the inside of the body.

Laparotomy. An operation that opens up the abdomen.

Large Intestine. The part of the intestine that goes from the cecum to the rectum. The large intestine absorbs water from stool and changes it from a liquid to a solid form. The large intestine is 5 feet long and includes the appendix, cecum, colon, and rectum. Also called colon.

Lavage. A cleaning of the stomach and colon. Uses a special drink and enemas. *See also* Bowel Prep.

Laxatives. Medicines to relieve long-term constipation. Used only if other methods fail. Also called cathartics.

Lazy Colon. *See* Atonic Colon.

Levator Syndrome. Feeling of fullness in the anus and rectum with occasional pain. Caused by muscle spasms.

Lithotripsy, Extracorporeal Shock Wave (ESWL). A method of breaking up bile stones and gallstones. Uses a specialized tool and shock waves.

Liver. The largest organ in the body. The liver carries out many important functions, such as making bile, changing food into energy, and cleaning alcohol and poisons from the blood.

Liver Enzyme Tests. Blood tests that look at how well the liver and biliary system are working. Also called liver function tests.

Liver Function Tests. *See* Liver Enzyme Tests.

Lower Esophageal Ring. An abnormal ring of tissue that may partially block the lower esophagus. Also called Schatzki's ring.

Lower Esophageal Sphincter. The muscle between the esophagus and stomach. When a person swallows, this muscle relaxes to let food pass from the esophagus to the stomach. It stays closed at other times to keep stomach contents from flowing back into the esophagus.

Lower GI Series. X-rays of the rectum, colon, and lower part of the small intestine. A barium enema is given first. Barium coats the organs so they will show up on the x-ray. Also called barium enema x-ray.

M

Magnetic Resonance Imaging (MRI). A test that takes pictures of the soft tissues in the body. The pictures are clearer than x-rays.

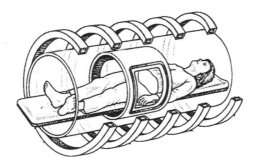

Figure 39.5. *Magnetic Resonance Imaging (MRI).*

Malabsorption Syndromes. Conditions that happen when the small intestine cannot absorb nutrients from foods.

Mallory-Weiss Tear. A tear in the lower end of the esophagus. Caused by severe vomiting. Common in alcoholics.

Malnutrition. A condition caused by not eating enough food or not eating a balanced diet.

Manometry. Tests that measure muscle pressure and movements in the GI tract. *See also* Esophageal Manometry and Rectal Manometry.

Meckel's Diverticulum. A birth defect in which a small sac forms in the ileum.

Megacolon. A huge, swollen colon. Results from severe constipation. In children, megacolon is more common in boys than girls. *See also* Hirschsprung's Disease.

Melena. Blood in the stool.

Ménétrier's Disease. A long-term disorder that causes large, coiled folds in the stomach. Also called giant hypertrophic gastritis.

Metabolism. The way cells change food into energy after food is digested and absorbed into the blood.

Motility. The movement of food through the digestive tract.

Motility Disorders. *See* Functional Disorders.

Mucosal Protective Drugs. Medicines that protect the stomach lining from acid. Examples are sucralfate (Carafate®), misoprostol (Cytotec®), antacids (Mylanta® and Maalox®), and bismuth subsalicylate (Pepto-Bismol®).

Mucous Colitis. *See* Irritable Bowel Syndrome.

Mucosal Lining. The lining of GI tract organs that makes mucus.

N

Nausea. The feeling of wanting to throw up (vomit).

Necrosis. Dead tissue that surrounds healthy tissue in the body.

Necrotizing Enterocolitis. A condition in which part of the tissue in the intestines is destroyed. Occurs mainly in under-weight newborn babies. A temporary ileostomy may be necessary.

Neonatal Hepatitis. Irritation of the liver with no known cause. Occurs in newborn babies. Symptoms include jaundice and liver cell changes.

Neoplasm. New and abnormal growth of tissue that may or may not cause cancer. Also called tumor.

Nissen Fundoplication. An operation to sew the top of the stomach (fundus) around the esophagus. Used to stop stomach contents from flowing back into the esophagus (reflux) and to repair a hiatal hernia.

Nontropical Sprue. *See* Celiac Disease.

Nonulcer Dyspepsia. Constant pain or discomfort in the upper GI tract. Symptoms include burning, nausea, and bloating, but no ulcer. Possibly caused by muscle spasms.

Norwalk Virus. A virus that may cause GI infection and diarrhea. *See also* Gastroenteritis.

Nutcracker Syndrome. Abnormal muscle tightening in the esophagus.

O

Obstruction. A blockage in the GI tract that prevents the flow of liquids or solids.

Occult Bleeding. Blood in stool that is not visible to the naked eye. May be a sign of disease such as diverticulosis or colorectal cancer.

Oral Dissolution Therapy. A method of dissolving cholesterol gallstones. The patient takes the oral medications chenodiol (Chenix®) and ursodiol (Actigall®). These medicines are most often used for people who cannot have an operation.

Ostomate. A person who has an ostomy. Called ostomist in some countries.

Ostomy. An operation that makes it possible for stool to leave the body through an opening made in the abdomen. An ostomy is necessary when part or all of the intestines are removed. Colostomy and ileostomy are types of ostomy.

P

Pancreas. A gland that makes enzymes for digestion and the hormone insulin.

Pancreatitis. Irritation of the pancreas that can make it stop working. Most often caused by gallstones or alcohol abuse.

Papillary Stenosis. A condition in which the openings of the bile ducts and pancreatic ducts narrow.

Parenteral Nutrition. A way to provide a liquid food mixture through a special tube in the chest. Also called hyperalimentation or total parenteral nutrition.

Parietal Cells. Cells in the stomach wall that make hydrochloric acid.

Pediatric Gastroenterologist. A doctor who treats children with digestive diseases.

Pepsin. An enzyme made in the stomach that breaks down proteins.

Peptic. Related to the stomach and the duodenum, where pepsin is present.

Peptic Ulcer. A sore in the lining of the esophagus, stomach, or duodenum. Usually caused by the bacterium *Helicobacter pylori*. An ulcer in the stomach is a gastric ulcer; an ulcer in the duodenum is a duodenal ulcer.

Percutaneous. Passing through the skin.

Percutaneous Transhepatic Cholangiography. X-rays of the gallbladder and bile ducts. A dye is injected through the abdomen to make the organs show up on the x-ray.

Perforated Ulcer. An ulcer that breaks through the wall of the stomach or the duodenum. Causes stomach contents to leak into the abdominal cavity.

Perforation. A hole in the wall of an organ.

Perianal. The area around the anus.

Perineal. Related to the perineum.

Perineum. The area between the anus and the sex organs.

Peristalsis. A wavelike movement of muscles in the GI tract. Peristalsis moves food and liquid through the GI tract.

Peritoneum. The lining of the abdominal cavity.

Peritonitis. Infection of the peritoneum.

Pernicious Anemia. Anemia caused by a lack of vitamin B_{12}. The body needs B_{12} to make red blood cells.

Peutz-Jeghers Syndrome. An inherited condition. Many polyps grow in the intestine. There is little risk of cancer.

Pharynx. The space behind the mouth. Serves as a passage for food from the mouth to the esophagus and for air from the nose and mouth to the larynx.

Polyp. Tissue bulging from the surface of an organ. Although these growths are not normal, they often are not cause for concern. However, people who have polyps in the colon may have an increased risk of colorectal cancer.

Polyposis. The presence of many polyps.

Porphyria. A group of rare, inherited blood disorders. When a person has porphyria, cells fail to change chemicals (porphyrins) to the substance (heme) that gives blood its color. Porphyrins then build up in the body. They show up in large amounts in stool and urine, causing the urine to be colored blue. They cause a number of problems, including strange behavior.

Portal Hypertension. High blood pressure in the portal vein. This vein carries blood into the liver. Portal hypertension is caused by a blood clot. This is a common complication of cirrhosis.

Portal Vein. The large vein that carries blood from the intestines and spleen to the liver.

Portosystemic Shunt. An operation to create an opening between the portal vein and other veins around the liver.

Postcholecystectomy Syndrome. A condition that occurs after gallbladder removal. The muscle between the gallbladder and the small intestine does not work properly, causing pain, nausea, and indigestion. Also called biliary dyskinesia.

Postgastrectomy Syndrome. A condition that occurs after an operation to remove the stomach (gastrectomy). *See also* Dumping Syndrome.

Postvagotomy Stasis. Delayed stomach emptying. Occurs after surgery on the vagus nerve.

Pouch. A special bag worn over a stoma to collect stool. Also called an ostomy appliance.

Primary Biliary Cirrhosis. A chronic liver disease. Slowly destroys the bile ducts in the liver. This prevents release of bile. Long-term irritation of the liver may cause scarring and cirrhosis in later stages of the disease.

Primary Sclerosing Cholangitis. Irritation, scarring, and narrowing of the bile ducts inside and outside the liver. Bile builds up in the liver and may damage its cells. Many people with this condition also have ulcerative colitis.

Proctalgia Fugax. Intense pain in the rectum that occasionally happens at night. Caused by muscle spasms around the anus.

Proctectomy. An operation to remove the rectum.

Proctitis. Irritation of the rectum.

Proctocolectomy. An operation to remove the colon and rectum. Also called coloproctectomy.

Proctocolitis. Irritation of the colon and rectum.

Proctologist. A doctor who specializes in disorders of the anus and rectum.

Proctoscope. A short, rigid metal tube used to look into the rectum and anus.

Proctoscopy. Looking into the rectum and anus with a proctoscope.

Proctosigmoiditis. Irritation of the rectum and the sigmoid colon.

Proctosigmoidoscopy. An endoscopic examination of the rectum and sigmoid colon. *See also* Endoscopy.

Prokinetic Drugs. Medicines that cause muscles in the GI tract to move food. An example is cisapride (Propulsid®).

Prolapse. A condition that occurs when a body part slips from its normal position.

Protcin. One of the three main classes of food. Protein is found in meat, eggs, and beans. The stomach and small intestine break down proteins into amino acids. The blood absorbs amino acids and uses them to build and mend cells. *See also* Amino Acids.

Proton Pump Inhibitors. Medicines that stop the stomach's acid pump. Examples are omeprazole (Prilosec®) and lansoprazole (Prevacid®).

Prune Belly Syndrome. A condition of newborn babies. The baby has no abdominal muscles, so the stomach looks like a shriveled prune. Also called Eagle-Barrett syndrome.

Pruritus Ani. Itching around the anus.

Pseudomembranous Colitis. Severe irritation of the colon. Caused by *Clostridium difficile* bacteria. Occurs after taking oral antibiotics, which kill bacteria that normally live in the colon.

Pyloric Sphincter. The muscle between the stomach and the small intestine.

Pyloric Stenosis. A narrowing of the opening between the stomach and the small intestine.

Pyloroplasty. An operation to widen the opening between the stomach and the small intestine. This allows stomach contents to pass more freely from the stomach.

Pylorus. The opening from the stomach into the top of the small intestine (duodenum).

R

Radiation Colitis. Damage to the colon from radiation therapy.

Radiation Enteritis. Damage to the small intestine from radiation therapy.

Radionuclide Scans. Tests to find GI bleeding. Radioactive material is injected to highlight organs on a special camera. Also called scintigraphy.

Rapid Gastric Emptying. *See* Dumping Syndrome.

Rectal Manometry. A test that uses a thin tube and balloon to measure pressure and movements of the rectal and anal sphincter muscles. Usually used to diagnose chronic constipation and fecal incontinence.

Rectal Prolapse. A condition in which the rectum slips so that it protrudes from the anus.

Rectum. The lower end of the large intestine, leading to the anus.

Reflux. A condition that occurs when gastric juices or small amounts of food from the stomach flow back into the esophagus and mouth. Also called regurgitation.

Reflux Esophagitis. Irritation of the esophagus because stomach contents flow back into the esophagus.

Regional Enteritis. *See* Crohn's Disease.

Regurgitation. *See* Reflux.

Retching. Dry vomiting.

Rotavirus. The most common cause of infectious diarrhea in the United States, especially in children under age 2.

Rupture. A break or tear in any organ or soft tissue.

S

Saliva. A mixture of water, protein, and salts that makes food easy to swallow and begins digestion.

Salmonella. A bacterium that may cause intestinal infection and diarrhea. *See also* Gastroenteritis.

Sarcoidosis. A condition that causes small, fleshy swellings in the liver, lungs, and spleen.

Schatzki's Ring. *See* Lower Esophageal Ring.

Scintigraphy. *See* Radionuclide Scans.

Sclerotherapy. A method of stopping upper GI bleeding. A needle is inserted through an endoscope to bring hardening agents to the place that is bleeding.

Secretin. A hormone made in the duodenum. Causes the stomach to make pepsin, the liver to make bile, and the pancreas to make a digestive juice.

Segmentation. The process by which muscles in the intestines move food and wastes through the body.

Shigellosis. Infection with the bacterium *Shigella*. Usually causes a high fever, acute diarrhea, and dehydration. *See also* Gastroenteritis.

Short Bowel Syndrome. Problems related to absorbing nutrients after removal of part of the small intestine. Symptoms include diarrhea, weakness, and weight loss. Also called short gut syndrome.

Short Gut Syndrome. *See* Short Bowel Syndrome.

Shwachman's Syndrome. A digestive and respiratory disorder of children. Certain digestive enzymes are missing and white blood cells are few. Symptoms may include diarrhea and short stature.

Sigmoid Colon. The lower part of the colon that empties into the rectum.

Sigmoidoscopy. Looking into the sigmoid colon and rectum with a flexible or rigid tube, called a sigmoidoscope.

Sitz Bath. A special plastic tub. A person sits in a few inches of warm water to help relieve discomfort of hemorrhoids or anal fissures.

Small Bowel Enema. X-rays of the small intestine taken as barium liquid passes through the organ. Also called small bowel follow-through. *See also* Lower GI Series.

Small Bowel Follow-Through. *See* Small Bowel Enema.

Small Intestine. Organ where most digestion occurs. It measures about 20 feet and includes the duodenum, jejunum, and ileum.

Solitary Rectal Ulcer. A rare type of ulcer in the rectum. May develop because of straining to have a bowel movement.

Somatostatin. A hormone in the pancreas. Somatostatin helps tell the body when to make the hormones insulin, glucagon, gastrin, secretin, and renin.

Spasms. Muscle movements such as those in the colon that cause pain, cramps, and diarrhea.

Spastic Colon. *See* Irritable Bowel Syndrome (IBS).

Sphincter. A ring-like band of muscle that opens and closes an opening in the body. An example is the muscle between the esophagus and the stomach known as the lower esophageal sphincter.

Sphincter of Oddi. The muscle between the common bile duct and pancreatic ducts.

Spleen. The organ that cleans blood and makes white blood cells. White blood cells attack bacteria and other foreign cells.

Splenic Flexure Syndrome. A condition that occurs when air or gas collects in the upper parts of the colon. Causes pain in the upper left abdomen. The pain often moves to the left chest and may be confused with heart problems.

Squamous Epithelium. Tissue in an organ such as the esophagus. Consists of layers of flat, scaly cells.

Steatorrhea. A condition in which the body cannot absorb fat. Causes a buildup of fat in the stool and loose, greasy, and foul bowel movements.

Steatosis. *See* Fatty Liver.

Stoma. An opening in the abdomen that is created by an operation (ostomy). Must be covered at all times by a bag that collects stool.

Stomach. The organ between the esophagus and the small intestine. The stomach is where digestion of protein begins.

Stomach Ulcer. An open sore in the lining of the stomach. Also called gastric ulcer.

Stool. The solid wastes that pass through the rectum as bowel movements. Stools are undigested foods, bacteria, mucus, and dead cells. Also called feces.

Stress Ulcer. An upper GI ulcer from physical injury such as surgery, major burns, or critical head injury.

Stricture. The abnormal narrowing of a body opening. Also called stenosis. *See also* Esophageal Stricture and Pyloric Stenosis.

T

Tenesmus. Straining to have a bowel movement. May be painful and continue for a long time without result.

Total Parenteral Nutrition (TPN). *See* Parenteral Nutrition.

Tracheoesophageal Fistula (TEF). A condition that occurs when there is a gap between the upper and lower segments of the esophagus. Food and saliva cannot pass through.

Transverse Colon. The part of the colon that goes across the abdomen from right to left.

Travelers' Diarrhea. An infection caused by unclean food or drink. Often occurs during travel outside one's own country. *See also* Gastroenteritis.

Triple-Therapy. A combination of three medicines used to treat *Helicobacter pylori* infection and ulcers. Drugs that stop the body from making acid are often added to relieve symptoms.

Tropical Sprue. A condition of unknown cause. Abnormalities in the lining of the small intestine prevent the body from absorbing food normally.

Tube Feeding. *See* Enteral Nutrition.

U

Ulcer. A sore on the skin surface or on the stomach lining.

Ulcerative Colitis. A serious disease that causes ulcers and irritation in the inner lining of the colon and rectum. See also Inflammatory Bowel Disease (IBD).

Upper GI Endoscopy. Looking into the esophagus, stomach, and duodenum with an endoscope. *See also* Endoscopy.

Upper GI Series. X-rays of the esophagus, stomach, and duodenum. The patient swallows barium first. Barium makes the organs show up on x-rays. Also called barium meal.

Urea Breath Test. A test used to detect *Helicobacter pylori* infection. The test measures breath samples for urease, an enzyme *H. pylori* makes.

V

Vagotomy. An operation to cut the vagus nerve. This causes the stomach to make less acid.

Vagus Nerve. The nerve in the stomach that controls the making of stomach acid.

Valve. A fold in the lining of an organ that prevents fluid from flowing backward.

Varices. Stretched veins such as those that form in the esophagus from cirrhosis.

VATER. A word made from the first letters of a group of birth defects. It is used when all of these birth defects affect the same child. The birth defects are: **V**ertebral defects, **A**nal malformations, **T**racheoesophageal fistula, **E**sophageal atresia, and **R**enal defects.

Villi. The tiny, fingerlike projections on the surface of the small intestine. Villi help absorb nutrients.

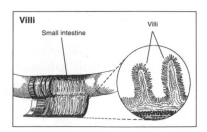

Figure 39.6. Villi, located in the small intestine, help absorb nutrients as food is digested.

Viral Hepatitis. Hepatitis caused by a virus. Five different viruses (A, B, C, D, and E) most commonly cause this form of hepatitis. Other rare viruses may also cause hepatitis. *See* Hepatitis.

Volvulus. A twisting of the stomach or large intestine. May be caused by the stomach being in the wrong position, a foreign substance, or abnormal joining of one part of the stomach or intestine to another. Volvulus can lead to blockage, perforation, peritonitis, and poor blood flow.

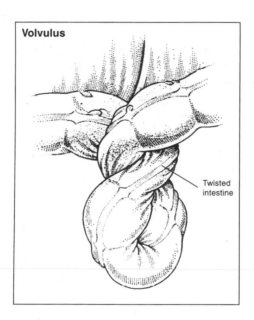

Volvulus

Twisted
intestine

Figure 39.7. Volvulus is a twisting of the stomach or large intestine.

Vomiting. The release of stomach contents through the mouth.

W

Watermelon Stomach. Parallel red sores in the stomach that look like the stripes on a watermelon. Frequently seen with cirrhosis.

Wilson's Disease. An inherited disorder. Too much copper builds up in the liver and is slowly released into other parts of the body. The overload can cause severe liver and brain damage if not treated with medication.

X

Xerostomia. Dry mouth. The condition can be caused by a number of things, including rheumatoid arthritis, diabetes, kidney failure, infection with HIV (the virus that causes AIDS), drugs used to treat depression, and radiation treatment for mouth or throat cancer.

Z

Zenker's Diverticulum. Pouches in the esophagus from increased pressure in and around the esophagus.

Zollinger-Ellison Syndrome. A group of symptoms that occur when a tumor called a gastrinoma forms in the pancreas. The tumor, which may cause cancer, releases large amounts of the hormone gastrin. The gastrin causes too much acid in the duodenum, resulting in ulcers, bleeding, and perforation.

Chapter 40

Directory of Digestive Diseases Organizations

Alagille Syndrome Alliance
10630 SW Garden Park Place
Tigard, OR 97223
Phone: (503) 639-6217
E-mail: cchahn@worldnet.att.net
Internet: http://www.athenet.net/~luxhoj/Alagillesyndrome.html

   Mission: Provides a support network for children, their parents, and others with Alagille syndrome.

American Celiac Society—Dietary Support Coalition
58 Musano Court
West Orange, NJ 07052
Phone: (201) 325-8837
Fax: (201) 669-8808

   Mission: Provides practical assistance to members and individuals with celiac disease and information about the disease to the public.

American College of Gasteroenterology
4900–B South 31st Street
Arlington, VA 22206-1656
Phone: (703) 820-7400

   This chapter contains information about resources compiled from that National Institute of Digestive and Digestive and Kidney Diseases and other organizations; contact information verified and updated in June 1999.

Fax: (703) 931-4520
Internet: http://www.acg.gi.org

Mission: Serves clinical and scientific information needs of member physicians and surgeons, who specialize in digestive and related disorders. Emphasis is on scholarly practice, teaching, and research.

American Gastroenterological Association
National Office
7910 Woodmont Avenue, 7th Floor
Bethesda, MD 20814
Phone: (301) 645-2055
Fax: (301) 654-3890
E-mail: kallen@gastro.org
Internet: http://www.gastro.org

Mission: Fosters the development and application of the science of gastroenterology by providing leadership and aid, including patient care, research, teaching, continuing education, scientific communication, and matters of national health policy pertaining to gastroenterology.

American Liver Foundation (ALF)
75 Maiden Lane, Suite 603
New York, NY 10038
Phone: (800) 465-4837
Fax: (201) 256-3214 fax
E-mail: webmail@liverfoundation.org
Internet: http://www.liverfoundation.org

Mission: Promotes awareness and supports research on liver disease; disseminates information about liver wellness, liver disease, and prevention of liver disease with audiovisual and printed materials, seminars, and training programs; promotes organ donation; encourages vaccination against hepatitis B; serves as trustee of transplant funds; and offers support groups through local chapters.

American Pancreatic Association
c/o Howard A. Reber, MD
UCLA School of Medicine
10833 LeConte Avenue
77-256 CHS
Los Angeles, CA 90024-6904

Phone: (310) 825-4976
Fax: (310) 206-2472
E-mail: hreber@surgery.medsch.ucla.edu

Mission: Provides a forum for the presentation of scientific research related to the pancreas.

American Porphyria Foundation
P.O. Box 22712
Houston, TX 77227
Phone: (713) 266-9617
Internet: http://www.cnterprise.net/apf/index.html

Mission: Advances awareness, research, and treatment of the porphyrias; provides self-help services for members; and provides referrals to porphyria treatment specialists.

American Pseudo-obstruction and Hirschsprung's Disease Society Inc. (APHS)
158 Pleasant Street
North Andover, MA 01845-2797
Phone: (508) 685-4477
Fax: (508) 685-4488
E-mail: aphs@tiac.net
Internet: http://www.tiac.net/users/aphs/

Mission: Promotes public awareness of gastrointestinal motility disorders, in particular intestinal pseudo-obstruction and Hirschsprung's disease; provides education and support to individuals and families of children who have been diagnosed with these disorders through person-to-person contact, publications, and educational symposia; and encourages and supports medical research in the area of gastrointestinal motility disorders.

American Society of Adults with Pseudo-Obstruction Inc. (ASAP)
International Corporate Headquarters
19 Carroll Road
Woburn, MA 01801
Phone: (781) 935-9776
Fax: (781) 933-4151
E-mail: asapgi@sprynet.com

Mission: Educates the general public and medical community about chronic intestinal pseudo-obstruction (CIP) and other related digestive motility disorders; serves as an integral resource of information for patients of all ages with CIP and related digestive motility disorders, their families, and members of the medical community; provides support and networking for members of ASAP and family members, including a special young adult network; supplies information concerning social security disability, doctor-patient relationships, coping with a rare disease, living as a caregiver of a person suffering from CIP and other related digestive motility disorders; also provides literature on other patient concerns. ASAP maintains a continually updated reference library of pertinent articles from recognized international medical journals that is available to its members. The organization has a prestigious Medical Advisory Board consisting of prominent physicians in the field of gastroenterology and a certified nutrition consultant. The international organization offers both general membership (including infants, children, teenagers, adults, families, and friends) and professional enrollment available to physicians, nurses, scientists, researchers, and other members of the medical community.

American Society for Gastrointestinal Endoscopy
13 Elm Street
Manchester, MA 01944-1314
Phone: (978) 526-4018
Fax: (978) 526-4018
E-mail: asge@idt.mail.net
Internet: http://www.asge.org

Mission: Provides information, training, and practice guidelines about gastrointestinal endoscopic techniques.

American Society for Parenteral and Enteral Nutrition
8630 Fenton Street, Suite 412
Silver Spring, MD 20910-3805
Phone: (301) 587-6315
Fax: (301) 587-2365
E-mail: aspen@nutr.org
Internet: http://www.clinnutr.org

Mission: Offers information and continuing medical education to professionals involved in the care of parenterally and enterally fed patients.

American Society of Abdominal Surgeons
675 Main Street
Melrose, MA 02176-3195
Phone: (781) 665-6102
Fax: (781) 655-4127
E-mail: office@abdominalsurg.org

Mission: Sponsors extensive continuing education program for physicians in the field of abdominal surgery and maintains a library.

American Society of Colon and Rectal Surgeons
85 West Algonquin Road, Suite 550
Arlington Heights, IL 60005
Phone: (847) 290-9184
Fax: (847) 290-9273
E-mail: ascrs@fascrs.org
Internet: http://www.fascrs.org

Mission: Serves as an information network for surgeons specializing in the diagnosis and treatment of colorectal disorders.

Celiac Disease Foundation (CDF)
13251 Ventura Boulevard, #3
Studio City, CA 91604-1838
Phone: (818) 990-2354
Fax: (818) 990-2379

Mission: Provides services and support to people with celiac disease and dermatitis herpetiformis, through programs of awareness, education, advocacy, and research; telephone information and referral services; medical advisory board; and special educational seminars and quarterly meetings.

Celiac Sprue Association/USA Inc.
P.O. Box 31700
Omaha, NE 68131-0700
Phone: (402) 558-0600
Fax: (402) 558-1347
E-mail: celiacs@csaceliacs.org
Internet: http://www.csaceliacs.org/

Mission: Provides information and referral services for persons with celiac sprue and dermatitis herpetiformis and parents of celiac children. Made up of six regions in the United States with 42 chapters and 78 resource units.

Children's Motility Disorder Foundation
PO Box 54869
Atlanta, GA 30308
Phone: (800) 809-9492
Fax: (404) 529-9202
E-mail: cmdf@motility.org
Internet: http://www.motility.org

Mission: Works to increase awareness of pediatric motility disorders in the general public and among the physicians most likely to encounter children suffering from these conditions, such as pediatricians and family practice doctors. Supports medical research regarding the causes, treatment, and potentially life-threatening disorders.

Crohn's and Colitis Foundation of America Inc.
386 Park Avenue South, 17th floor
New York, NY 10016-8804
Phone: (800) 932-2423 or (212) 685-3440
Fax: (212) 779-4098
E-mail: info@ccfa.org
Internet: http://www.ccfa.org

Mission: Supports basic and clinical research on a cure and treatment for Crohn's disease and ulcerative colitis; conducts professional education activities; produces public service programs and a wide variety of literature about inflammatory bowel disease for patients and their families, professionals, and the public; and sponsors 70 chapters and affiliates.

Cyclic Vomiting Syndrome Association (CVSA)
3707 Cedar Hill Rd NW
Canal Winchester, Ohio 43110
Phone: (614) 837-2586
Fax: (614) 837-6543
E-mail: drwaites@infinet.com
Internet: http://www.beaker.iupui.edu/cvsa

Mission: Provides opportunities for patients, families, and professionals to offer and receive support and share knowledge about cyclic vomiting syndrome; actively promotes and facilitates medical research; increases worldwide public and professional awareness; and serves as a resource center for information.

Food Allergy Network
10400 Eaton Place, Suite 107
Fairfax, VA 22030-2208
Phone: (703) 691-3179
Fax: (703) 691-2713
E-mail: fan@worldweb.net
Internet: http://www.foodallergy.org

Mission: Increases public awareness about food allergies and anaphylaxis and helps families living with food allergies. Provides education, emotional support, and coping strategies to patients, and serves as the communication link between the food industry, the Government, the airline industry, and the food-allergic consumer.

Gastro-Intestinal Research Foundation
70 East Lake Street, Suite 1015
Chicago, IL 60601-5907
Phone: (312) 332-1350
Fax: (312) 332-4757

Mission: Supports research and training programs at the University of Chicago Medical Center, Section of Gastroenterology; sponsors educational activities for the public.

Gluten Intolerance Group of North America
5110 10th Avenue, SW
Suite A
Seattle, WA 98166-1820
Phone: (206) 246-6652
Fax: (206) 246-6531
E-mail: gig@accessone.com

Mission: Provides instructional and general information materials, counseling, and access to gluten-free products and ingredients to persons with celiac sprue and their families; operates telephone information and referral service; conducts educational seminars for health professionals; conducts and supports research; and offers leadership and assistance to 14 affiliates and local member contacts.

The Hemochromatosis Foundation Inc.

P.O. Box 8569
Albany, NY 12208-2569
Phone: (518) 489-0972
Fax: (518) 489-0227
Internet: http://www.hemochromatosis.org

Mission: Provides information to the public, families, and professionals about hereditary hemochromatosis (HH); conducts and raises funds for research; encourages early screening for HH; holds symposiums and meetings; and offers genetic counseling along with support for patients and professionals.

Hepatitis B Coalition

Immunization Action Coalition
1573 Selby Avenue
St. Paul, MN 55104
Phone: (651) 647-9009
Fax: (651) 647-9131
E-mail: admin@immunize.org
Internet: http://www.immunize.org

Mission: Works to prevent transmission of hepatitis B in high-risk groups; to achieve vaccination of all infants, children, and adolescents; and to promote education and treatment for the hepatitis B carrier.

Hepatitis B Foundation

700 East Butler Avenue
Doylestown, PA 18901-2697
Phone: (215) 489-4900
E-mail: info@hepb.org
Internet: http://www2.hepb.org/hepb/

Mission: Provides support and education to people affected by hepatitis B and dedicates itself to eliminating hepatitis B through community education and cure research programs.

Hepatitis Foundation International (HFI)

30 Sunrise Terrace
Cedar Grove, NJ 07009-1423
Phone: (973) 239-1035 or (800) 891-0707
Fax: (973) 857-5044

E-mail: mail@hepfi.org
Internet: http://www.hepfi.org

Mission: Fosters worldwide awareness about the prevention, diagnosis, and treatment of viral hepatitis; provides patient and professional education programs; distributes publications; and supports research. A unique service is the Patient Advocacy/Information Telecommunications System, a phone support network that enables patients to talk to others with similar concerns.

International Foundation for Functional Gastrointestinal Disorders (IFFGD)

P.O. Box 17864
Milwaukee, WI 53217
Phone: (888) 964-2001 or (414) 964-1799
Fax: (414) 964-7176
E-mail: iffgd@iffgd.org
Internet: http://www.iffgd.org

Mission: Provides support and educational information for people affected by functional gastrointestinal disorders, including irritable bowel syndrome (IBS), constipation, diarrhea, pain, and incontinence.

Intestinal Disease Foundation, Inc.

1323 Forbes Avenue, Suite 200
Pittsburgh, PA 15219
Phone: (412) 261-5888
Fax: (412) 471-2722
E-mail: lschorr@aol.com

Mission: Provides one-on-one telephone support, educational programs and materials, and self-help groups for people with irritable bowel syndrome (IBS) and inflammatory bowel diseases, primarily in the Pennsylvania-Ohio-West Virginia area; sponsors medical seminars and educational meetings; and provides a speakers' bureau, research updates, and physician referral lists.

Iron Overload Diseases Association Inc.

433 Westward Drive
North Palm Beach, FL 33408
Phone: (561) 840-8512
Fax: (561) 842-9881

E-mail: iod@ironoverload.org
Internet: http://www.ironoverload.org

Mission: Conducts professional education symposiums and exhibits at medical meetings; serves and counsels hemochromatosis patients and families; offers doctor referrals; promotes patient advocacy concerning insurance, Medicare, blood banks, and the Food and Drug Administration; encourages research; maintains international consortium; offers public information through the media; develops chapters and self-help groups; and sponsors annual symposiums and annual IOD Awareness Week.

National Association For Continence (NAFC) (formerly Help for Incontinent People (HIP))
P.O. Box 8310
Spartanburg, SC 29305-8310
Phone: (800) BLADDER or (864) 579-7900
Fax: (864) 579-7902
Internet: http://www.nafc.org/

Mission: A leading source of education, advocacy, and support to the public and to the health profession about the causes, prevention, diagnosis, treatments, and management alternatives for incontinence.

National Center for Nutrition and Dietetics (NCND) of The American Dietetic Association
216 West Jackson Boulevard, Suite 800
Chicago, IL 60606-6995
Consumer Nutrition Hotline: (800) 366-1655
Internet: http://www.eatright.org

Mission: Provides consumers with direct and immediate access to reliable nutrition information. Callers may speak to a registered dietitian, may listen to regularly updated nutrition messages in English or Spanish, or may be referred to a dietitian in their local area.

National Digestive Diseases Information Clearinghouse
2 Information Way
Bethesda, MD 20892-3570
E-mail: nddic@info.niddk.nih.gov

Mission: A service of the National Institute of Diabetes and Digestive and Kidney Diseases (NIDDK). The NIDDK is part of the

National Institutes of Health under the U.S. Public Health Service. Established in 1980, the clearinghouse provides information about digestive diseases to people with digestive disorders and to their families, health care professionals, and the public. NDDIC answers inquiries; develops, reviews, and distributes publications; and works closely with professional and patient organizations and Government agencies to coordinate resources about digestive diseases.

National Organization for Rare Disorders Inc. (NORD®)

P.O. Box 8923
New Fairfield, CT 06812-8923
Phone: (800) 999-6673 or (203) 746-6518
Fax: (203) 746-6481
E-mail: orphan@nord-rdb.com
Internet: http://www.NORD-RDB.com/~orphan

Mission: Serves as a clearinghouse for information about rare disorders and brings together families with similar disorders for mutual support; fosters communication among rare disease voluntary agencies, government agencies, industry, scientific researchers, academic institutions, and concerned individuals; and encourages and promotes research and education on rare disorders and orphan drugs.

North American Society for Pediatric Gastroenterology and Nutrition

c/o SLACK, Inc.
6900 Grove Road
Thorofare, NJ 08086
Phone: (609) 848-1000
Fax: (609) 853-5274
E-mail: naspgn@slackinc.com
Internet: http://www.naspgn.org/

Mission: Promotes research and provides a forum for professionals in the areas of pediatric GI liver disease, gastroenterology, and nutrition. Associated with fellow organizations in Europe and Australia (ESPGAN, AUSPGAN).

The Oley Foundation Inc.

214 Hun Memorial, A-23
Albany Medical Center
Albany, NY 12208-3478

Phone: (800) 776-OLEY or (518) 262-5079
Fax: (518) 262-5528
E-mail: joan bishop@ccgateway.amc.edu
Internet: http://web.wizvax.net/oleyfdn/lifeline/95-010.htm

Mission: Promotes and advocates education and research in home parenteral and enteral nutrition; provides support and networking to patients through information clearinghouse and regional volunteer networks; sponsors meetings and conferences, including annual patient/clinician conference; maintains speakers' bureau; manages the North American Home Parenteral and Enteral Nutrition Patient Registry (formerly known as OASIS), a voluntary database of patient-outcome information from across the United States and Canada; and publishes annual summaries of results and basic statistics.

Pediatric/Adolescent Gastroesophageal Reflux Association Inc. (PAGER)
P.O. Box 1153
Germantown, MD 20875-1153
Phone: (301) 601-9541
E-mail: GERGROUP@aol.com
Internet: http://www.reflux.org

Mission: Gathers and disseminates information on pediatric gastroesophageal reflux and related disorders; provides support and education to patients, their families, and the public; promotes the general welfare of patients with gastroesophageal reflux and their families; and promotes public awareness of the condition.

Pediatric Crohn's & Colitis Association Inc.
P.O. Box 188
Newton, MA 02468
Phone: (617) 489-5854
E-mail: questions@pcca.hypermart.net
http://pcca.hypermart.net/

Mission: Focuses on all aspects of pediatric and adolescent Crohn's disease and ulcerative colitis, including medical, nutritional, psychological, and social factors. Activities include information sharing, educational forums, newsletters, a hospital outreach program, and support of research.

Pull-thru Network
4 Woody Lane
Westport, CT 06880
Phone: (203) 221-7530
E-mail: pullthrunw@aol.com
Internet: http://members.aol.com/pullthrunw/Pullthru.html

Mission: Provides emotional support and information to patients and families of children who have had or will have pull-through surgery to correct an imperforate anus or associated malformation, Hirschsprung's disease, or other fecal incontinence problems. Sponsors online discussion groups. A chapter of the United Ostomy Association.

The Simon Foundation for Continence
P.O. Box 815
Wilmette, IL 60091
Phone: (800) 23-SIMON or (847) 864-3913

Mission: Seeks to bring the topic of incontinence out of the closet and remove the associated stigma. Provides educational materials to patients, their families, and the health care professionals who provide patient care.

The Society for Surgery of the Alimentary Tract
13 Elm Street
Manchester, MA 01944
Phone: (978) 526-8330
Fax: (978) 526-4018
E-mail: ssat@prri.com
Internet: http://www.ssat.com/

Mission: Provides a forum for the exchange of information among physicians specializing in alimentary tract surgery.

Society of American Gastrointestinal Endoscopic Surgeons
2716 Ocean Park Boulevard, Suite 3000
Santa Monica, CA 90405
Phone: (301) 314-2404
Fax: (301) 314-2585
E-mail: sagesmail@aol.com
Internet: http://www.sages.org/sages.html

Mission: Encourages the study and practice of gastrointestinal endoscopy as an integral part of surgery.

Society of Gastroenterology Nurses and Associates, Inc.
401 North Michigan Avenue
Chicago, IL 60611-4267
Phone: (800) 245-7462 or (312) 321-5165
Fax: (312) 321-5194
E-mail: sgna@sba.com
Internet: http://www.sgna.org

Mission: Provides members with continuing education opportunities, practice and training guidelines, and information about trends and development in the field of gastroenterology.

TEF/VATER Support Network
15301 Grey Fox Road
Upper Marlboro, MD 20772
Phone: (301) 952-6837

Mission: Provides support to children and adults born with tracheoesophageal fistula (TEF), esophageal atresia, or VATER (V—vertebral defects, A—imperforate anus, TE—tracheoesophageal defects, R—radial and renal dysplasia).

United Network for Organ Sharing (UNOS)
1100 Boulders Parkway, Suite 500
P.O. Box 13770
Richmond, VA 23225-8770
Phone: (804) 24-DONOR or (804) 330-8500
Fax: (804) 330-8517
Internet: http://www.unos.org

Mission: Improves the effectiveness of human organ donation, procurement, distribution, and transplantation; and maintains scientific registry of transplant data.

United Ostomy Association Inc. (UOA)
19772 MacArthur Blvd., Suite 200
Irvine, CA 92612-2405
Phone: (800) 826-0826 or (714) 660-8624
Fax: (714) 660-9262

E-mail: uoa@deltanet.com
Home page: http://www.uoa.org

Mission: Produces and distributes materials about ostomy care and management; through trained UOA members, offers practical assistance and emotional support to ostomy patients; sponsors annual youth rally and State and regional conferences for local affiliates; and 650 chapters serve people locally.

Weight-control Information Network (WIN)
1 WIN Way
Bethesda, MD 20892-3665
Phone: (800) 946-8098 or (301) 984-7378
Fax: (301) 984-7196
E-mail: win@info.niddk.nih.gov
Internet: http://www.niddk.nih.gov

Mission: To address the health information needs of individuals through the production and dissemination of educational materials. In addition, WIN is developing communication strategies for a pilot program to encourage at-risk individuals to achieve and maintain a healthy weight by making changes in their lifestyle.

Wilson's Disease Association
4 Navaho Drive
Brookfield, CT 06810
Phone: (800) 399-0266 or (203) 775-9666
Fax: (203) 743-6196
E-mail: hasellner@worldnet.att.net
Internet: http://www.medhelp.org/wda/wil.htm

Mission: Serves as a communications and support network for individuals affected by Wilson's disease and related disorders of copper metabolism; distributes information to professionals and the public.

Wound, Ostomy, and Continence Nurses Society
1550 South Coast Highway, Suite 201
Laguna Beach, CA 92651
Phone: (888) 224-9626
Fax: (949) 376-3456
E-mail: membership@wocn.org
Internet: http://www.wocn.org

Mission: A professional nursing society that supports its members by promoting educational, clinical, and research opportunities to guide the delivery of health care to individuals with wounds, ostomies, and incontinence.

Index

Index

L

M

Health Reference Series
COMPLETE CATALOG

AIDS Sourcebook, 1st Edition

Basic Information about AIDS and HIV Infection, Featuring Historical and Statistical Data, Current Research, Prevention, and Other Special Topics of Interest for Persons Living with AIDS, Along with Source Listings for Further Assistance

Edited by Karen Bellenir and Peter D. Dresser. 831 pages. 1995. 0-7808-0031-1. $78.

"One strength of this book is its practical emphasis. The intended audience is the lay reader . . . useful as an educational tool for health care providers who work with AIDS patients. Recommended for public libraries as well as hospital or academic libraries that collect consumer materials." — *Bulletin of the MLA, Jan '96*

"This is the most comprehensive volume of its kind on an important medical topic. Highly recommended for all libraries." — *Reference Book Review, '96*

"Very useful reference for all libraries."
— *Choice, Oct '95*

"There is a wealth of information here that can provide much educational assistance. It is a must book for all libraries and should be on the desk of each and every congressional leader. Highly recommended."
— *AIDS Book Review Journal, Aug '95*

"Recommended for most collections."
— *Library Journal, Jul '95*

AIDS Sourcebook, 2nd Edition

Basic Consumer Health Information about Acquired Immune Deficiency Syndrome (AIDS) and Human Immunodeficiency Virus (HIV) Infection, Featuring Updated Statistical Data, Reports on Recent Research and Prevention Initiatives, and Other Special Topics of Interest for Persons Living with AIDS, Including New Antiretroviral Treatment Options, Strategies for Combating Opportunistic Infections, Information about Clinical Trials, and More; Along with a Glossary of Important Terms and Resource Listings for Further Help and Information

Edited by Karen Bellenir. 751 pages. 1999. 0-7808-0225-X. $78.

Allergies Sourcebook

Basic Information about Major Forms and Mechanisms of Common Allergic Reactions, Sensitivities, and Intolerances, Including Anaphylaxis, Asthma, Hives and Other Dermatologic Symptoms, Rhinitis, and Sinusitis, Along with Their Usual Triggers Like Animal Fur, Chemicals, Drugs, Dust, Foods, Insects, Latex, Pollen, and Poison Ivy, Oak, and Sumac; Plus Information on Prevention, Identification, and Treatment

Edited by Allan R. Cook. 611 pages. 1997. 0-7808-0036-2. $78.

Alternative Medicine Sourcebook

Basic Consumer Health Information about Alternatives to Conventional Medicine, Including Acupressure, Acupuncture, Aromatherapy, Ayurveda, Bioelectromagnetics, Environmental Medicine, Essence Therapy, Food and Nutrition Therapy, Herbal Therapy, Homeopathy, Imaging, Massage, Naturopathy, Reflexology, Relaxation and Meditation, Sound Therapy, Vitamin and Mineral Therapy, and Yoga, and More

Edited by Allan R. Cook. 737 pages. 1999. 0-7808-0200-4. $78.

Alzheimer's, Stroke & 29 Other Neurological Disorders Sourcebook, 1st Edition

Basic Information for the Layperson on 31 Diseases or Disorders Affecting the Brain and Nervous System, First Describing the Illness, Then Listing Symptoms, Diagnostic Methods, and Treatment Options, and Including Statistics on Incidences and Causes

Edited by Frank E. Bair. 579 pages. 1993. 1-55888-/48-2. $78.

"Nontechnical reference book that provides reader-friendly information."
— *Family Caregiver Alliance Update, Winter '96*

"Should be included in any library's patient education section." — *American Reference Books Annual, '94*

"Written in an approachable and accessible style. Recommended for patient education and consumer health collections in health science center and public libraries." — *Academic Library Book Review, Dec '93*

"It is very handy to have information on more than thirty neurological disorders under one cover, and there is no recent source like it." — *RQ, Fall '93*

Alzheimer's Disease Sourcebook, 2nd Edition

Basic Consumer Health Information about Alzheimer's Disease, Related Disorders, and Other Dementias, Including Multi-Infarct Dementia, AIDS-Related Dementia, Alcoholic Dementia, Huntington's Disease, Delirium, and Confusional States; Along with Reports Detailing Current Research Efforts in Prevention and Treatment, Long-Term Care Issues, and Listings of Sources for Additional Help and Information

Edited by Karen Bellenir. 524 pages. 1999. 0-7808-0223-3. $78.

Arthritis Sourcebook

Basic Consumer Health Information about Specific Forms of Arthritis and Related Disorders, Including Rheumatoid Arthritis, Osteoarthritis, Gout, Polymyalgia Rheumatica, Psoriatic Arthritis, Spondyloarthropathies, Juvenile Rheumatoid Arthritis, and Juvenile Ankylosing Spondylitis; Along with Information about Medical, Surgical, and Alternative Treatment Options, and Including Strategies for Coping with Pain, Fatigue, and Stress

Edited by Allan R. Cook. 550 pages. 1998. 0-7808-0201-2. $78.

"... accessible to the layperson."
— *Reference and Research Book News, Feb '99*

Back & Neck Disorders Sourcebook

Basic Information about Disorders and Injuries of the Spinal Cord and Vertebrae, Including Facts on Chiropractic Treatment, Surgical Interventions, Paralysis, and Rehabilitation, Along with Advice for Preventing Back Trouble

Edited by Karen Bellenir. 548 pages. 1997. 0-7808-0202-0. $78.

"The strength of this work is its basic, easy-to-read format. Recommended."
— *Reference and User Services Quarterly, Winter '97*

Blood & Circulatory Disorders Sourcebook

Basic Information about Blood and Its Components, Anemias, Leukemias, Bleeding Disorders, and Circulatory Disorders, Including Aplastic Anemia, Thalassemia, Sickle-Cell Disease, Hemochromatosis, Hemophilia, Von Willebrand Disease, and Vascular Diseases; Along with a Special Section on Blood Transfusions and Blood Supply Safety, a Glossary, and Source Listings for Further Help and Information

Edited by Karen Bellenir and Linda M. Shin. 554 pages. 1998. 0-7808-0203-9. $78.

"Recent and recommended reference source."
— *Booklist, Feb '99*

"An important reference sourcebook written in simple language for everyday, non-technical users. "
— *Reviewer's Bookwatch, Jan '99*

Brain Disorders Sourcebook

Basic Consumer Health Information about Strokes, Epilepsy, Amyotrophic Lateral Sclerosis (ALS/Lou Gehrig's Disease), Parkinson's Disease, Brain Tumors, Cerebral Palsy, Headache, Tourette Syndrome, and More; Along with Statistical Data, Treatment and Rehabilitation Options, Coping Strategies, Reports on Current Research Initiatives, a Glossary, and Resource Listings for Additional Help and Information

Edited by Karen Bellenir. 481 pages. 1999. 0-7808-0229-2. $78.

Burns Sourcebook

Basic Consumer Health Information about Various Types of Burns and Scalds, Including Flame, Heat, Cold, Electrical, Chemical, and Sun Burns; Along with Information on Short-Term and Long-Term Treatments, Tissue Reconstruction, Plastic Surgery, Prevention Suggestions, and First Aid

Edited by Allan R. Cook. 604 pages. 1999. 0-7808-0204-7. $78.

Cancer Sourcebook, 1st Edition

Basic Information on Cancer Types, Symptoms, Diagnostic Methods, and Treatments, Including Statistics on Cancer Occurrences Worldwide and the Risks Associated with Known Carcinogens and Activities

Edited by Frank E. Bair. 932 pages. 1990. 1-55888-888-8. $78.

"Written in nontechnical language. Useful for patients, their families, medical professionals, and librarians."
— *Guide to Reference Books, '96*

"Designed with the non-medical professional in mind. Libraries and medical facilities interested in patient education should certainly consider adding the Cancer Sourcebook to their holdings. This compact collection of reliable information ... is an invaluable tool for helping patients and patients' families and friends to take the first steps in coping with the many difficulties of cancer."
— *Medical Reference Services Quarterly, Winter '91*

"Specifically created for the nontechnical reader ... an important resource for the general reader trying to understand the complexities of cancer."
— *American Reference Books Annual, '91*

"This publication's nontechnical nature and very comprehensive format make it useful for both the general public and undergraduate students."
— *Choice, Oct '90*

New Cancer Sourcebook, 2nd Edition

Basic Information about Major Forms and Stages of Cancer, Featuring Facts about Primary and Secondary Tumors of the Respiratory, Nervous, Lymphatic, Circulatory, Skeletal, and Gastrointestinal Systems, and Specific Organs; Statistical and Demographic Data; Treatment Options; and Strategies for Coping

Edited by Allan R. Cook. 1,313 pages. 1996. 0-7808-0041-9. $78.

"This book is an excellent resource for patients with newly diagnosed cancer and their families. The dialogue is simple, direct, and comprehensive. Highly recommended for patients and families to aid in their understanding of cancer and its treatment."
— *Booklist Health Sciences Supplement, Oct '97*

"The amount of factual and useful information is extensive. The writing is very clear, geared to general readers. Recommended for all levels."
— *Choice, Jan '97*

Cancer Sourcebook, 3rd Edition

Basic Consumer Health Information about Major Forms and Stages of Cancer, Featuring Facts about Primary and Secondary Tumors of the Respiratory, Nervous, Lymphatic, Circulatory, Skeletal, and Gastrointestinal Systems, and Specific Organs; Along with Statistical and Demographic Data, Treatment Options, Strategies for Coping, a Glossary, and a Directory of Sources for Additional Help and Information

Edited by Edward J. Prucha. 1,100 pages. 1999. 0-7808-0227-6. $78.

Cancer Sourcebook for Women, 1st Edition

Basic Information about Specific Forms of Cancer That Affect Women, Featuring Facts about Breast Cancer, Cervical Cancer, Ovarian Cancer, Cancer of the Uterus and Uterine Sarcoma, Cancer of the Vagina, and Cancer of the Vulva; Statistical and Demographic Data; Treatments, Self-Help Management Suggestions, and Current Research Initiatives

Edited by Allan R. Cook and Peter D. Dresser. 524 pages. 1996. 0-7808-0076-1. $78.

". . . written in easily understandable, non-technical language. Recommended for public libraries or hospital and academic libraries that collect patient education or consumer health materials."
— *Medical Reference Services Quarterly, Spring '97*

"Would be of value in a consumer health library. . . . written with the health care consumer in mind. Medical jargon is at a minimum, and medical terms are explained in clear, understandable sentences."
— *Bulletin of the MLA, Oct '96*

"The availability under one cover of all these pertinent publications, grouped under cohesive headings, makes this certainly a most useful sourcebook."
— *Choice, Jun '96*

"Presents a comprehensive knowledge base for general readers. Men and women both benefit from the gold mine of information nestled between the two covers of this book. Recommended."
— *Academic Library Book Review, Summer '96*

"This timely book is highly recommended for consumer health and patient education collections in all libraries."
— *Library Journal, Apr '96*

Cancer Sourcebook for Women, 2nd Edition

Basic Consumer Health Information about Specific Forms of Cancer That Affect Women, Including Cervical Cancer, Ovarian Cancer, Endometrial Cancer, Uterine Sarcoma, Vaginal Cancer, Vulvar Cancer, and Gestational Trophoblastic Tumor; and Featuring Statistical Information, Facts about Tests and Treatments, a Glossary of Cancer Terms, and an Extensive List of Additional Resources

Edited by Edward J. Prucha. 600 pages. 1999. 0-7808-0226-8. $78.

Cardiovascular Diseases & Disorders Sourcebook, 1st Edition

Basic Information about Cardiovascular Diseases and Disorders, Featuring Facts about the Cardiovascular System, Demographic and Statistical Data, Descriptions of Pharmacological and Surgical Interventions, Lifestyle Modifications, and a Special Section Focusing on Heart Disorders in Children

Edited by Karen Bellenir and Peter D. Dresser. 683 pages. 1995. 0-7808-0032-X. $78.

". . . comprehensive format provides an extensive overview on this subject."
— *Choice, Jun '96*

". . . an easily understood, complete, up-to-date resource. This well executed public health tool will make valuable information available to those that need it most, patients and their families. The typeface, sturdy non-reflective paper, and library binding add a feel of quality found wanting in other publications. Highly recommended for academic and general libraries. "
— *Academic Library Book Review, Summer '96*

Communication Disorders Sourcebook

Basic Information about Deafness and Hearing Loss, Speech and Language Disorders, Voice Disorders, Balance and Vestibular Disorders, and Disorders of Smell, Taste, and Touch

Edited by Linda M. Ross. 533 pages. 1996. 0-7808-0077-X. $78.

"This is skillfully edited and is a welcome resource for the layperson. It should be found in every public and medical library."
— *Booklist Health Sciences Supplement, Oct '97*

Congenital Disorders Sourcebook

Basic Information about Disorders Acquired during Gestation, Including Spina Bifida, Hydrocephalus, Cerebral Palsy, Heart Defects, Craniofacial Abnormalities, Fetal Alcohol Syndrome, and More, Along with Current Treatment Options and Statistical Data

Edited by Karen Bellenir. 607 pages. 1997. 0-7808-0205-5. $78.

"Recent and recommended reference source."
— *Booklist, Oct '97*

Consumer Issues in Health Care Sourcebook

Basic Information about Health Care Fundamentals and Related Consumer Issues, Including Exams and Screening Tests, Physician Specialties, Choosing a Doctor, Using Prescription and Over-the-Counter Medications Safely, Avoiding Health Scams, Managing Common Health Risks in the Home, Care Options for Chronically or Terminally Ill Patients, and a List of Resources for Obtaining Help and Further Information

Edited by Karen Bellenir. 618 pages. 1998. 0-7808-0221-7. $78.

"The editor has researched the literature from government agencies and others, saving readers the time and effort of having to do the research themselves. Recommended for public libraries."
— *Reference and Users Services Quarterly, Spring '99*

"Recent and recommended reference source."
— *Booklist, Dec '98*

Contagious & Non-Contagious Infectious Diseases Sourcebook

Basic Information about Contagious Diseases like Measles, Polio, Hepatitis B, and Infectious Mononucleosis, and Non-Contagious Infectious Diseases like Tetanus and Toxic Shock Syndrome, and Diseases Occurring as Secondary Infections Such as Shingles and Reye Syndrome, Along with Vaccination, Prevention, and Treatment Information, and a Section Describing Emerging Infectious Disease Threats

Edited by Karen Bellenir and Peter D. Dresser. 566 pages. 1996. 0-7808-0075-3. $78.

Death & Dying Sourcebook

Basic Consumer Health Information for the Layperson about End-of-Life Care and Related Ethical and Legal Issues, Including Chief Causes of Death, Autopsies, Pain Management for the Terminally Ill, Life Support Systems, Insurance, Euthanasia, Assisted Suicide, Hospice Programs, Living Wills, Funeral Planning, Counseling, Mourning, Organ Donation, and Physician Training; Along with Statistical Data, a Glossary, and Listings of Sources for Further Help and Information

Edited by Annemarie S. Muth. 641 pages. 1999. 0-7808-0230-6. $78.

Diabetes Sourcebook, 1st Edition

Basic Information about Insulin-Dependent and Noninsulin-Dependent Diabetes Mellitus, Gestational Diabetes, and Diabetic Complications, Symptoms, Treatment, and Research Results, Including Statistics on Prevalence, Morbidity, and Mortality, Along with Source Listings for Further Help and Information

Edited by Karen Bellenir and Peter D. Dresser. 827 pages. 1994. 1-55888-751-2. $78.

"... very informative and understandable for the layperson without being simplistic. It provides a comprehensive overview for laypersons who want a general understanding of the disease or who want to focus on various aspects of the disease." — *Bulletin of the MLA, Jan '96*

Diabetes Sourcebook, 2nd Edition

Basic Consumer Health Information about Type 1 Diabetes (Insulin-Dependent or Juvenile-Onset Diabetes), Type 2 (Noninsulin-Dependent or Adult-Onset Diabetes), Gestational Diabetes, and Related Disorders, Including Diabetes Prevalence Data, Management Issues, the Role of Diet and Exercise in Controlling Diabetes, Insulin and Other Diabetes Medicines, and Complications of Diabetes Such as Eye Diseases, Periodontal Disease, Amputation, and End-Stage Renal Disease; Along with Reports on Current Research Initiatives, a Glossary, and Resource Listings for Further Help and Information

Edited by Karen Bellenir. 688 pages. 1998. 0-7808-0224-1. $78.

"Recent and recommended reference source."
— *Booklist, Feb '99*

Diet & Nutrition Sourcebook, 1st Edition

Basic Information about Nutrition, Including the Dietary Guidelines for Americans, the Food Guide Pyramid, and Their Applications in Daily Diet, Nutritional Advice for Specific Age Groups, Current Nutritional Issues and Controversies, the New Food Label and How to Use It to Promote Healthy Eating, and Recent Developments in Nutritional Research

Edited by Dan R. Harris. 662 pages. 1996. 0-7808-0084-2. $78.

"Useful reference as a food and nutrition sourcebook for the general consumer."
— *Booklist Health Sciences Supplement, Oct '97*

"Recommended for public libraries and medical libraries that receive general information requests on nutrition. It is readable and will appeal to those interested in learning more about healthy dietary practices."
— *Medical Reference Services Quarterly, Fall '97*

Diet & Nutrition Sourcebook, 2nd Edition

Basic Consumer Health Information about Dietary Guidelines, Recommended Daily Intake Values, Vitamins, Minerals, Fiber, Fat, Weight Control, Dietary Supplements, and Food Additives; Along with Special Sections on Nutrition Needs throughout Life and Nutrition for People with Such Specific Medical Concerns as Allergies, High Blood Cholesterol, Hypertension, Diabetes, Celiac Disease, Seizure Disorders, Phenylketonuria (PKU), Cancer, and Eating Disorders, and Including Reports on Current Nutrition Research and Source Listings for Additional Help and Information

Edited by Karen Bellenir. 650 pages. 1999. 0-7808-0228-4. $78.

Digestive Diseases & Disorders Sourcebook

Basic Consumer Health Information about Diseases and Disorders that Impact the Upper and Lower Digestive System, Including Celiac Disease, Constipation, Crohn's Disease, Cyclic Vomiting Syndrome, Diarrhea, Diverticulosis and Diverticulitis, Gallstones, Heartburn, Hemorrhoids, Hernias, Indigestion (Dyspepsia), Irritable Bowel Syndrome, Lactose Intolerance, Ulcers, and More; Along with Information about Medications and Other Treatments, Tips for Maintaining a Healthy Digestive Tract, a Glossary, and Directory of Digestive Diseases Organizations

Edited by Karen Bellenir. 335 pages. 1999. 0-7808-0327-2. $48.

Disabilities Sourcebook

Basic Consumer Health Information about Physical and Psychiatric Disabilities, Including Descriptions of Major Causes of Disability, Assistive and Adaptive Aids, Workplace Issues, and Accessibility Concerns; Along with Information about the Americans with Disabilities Act, a Glossary, and Resources for Additional Help and Information

Edited by Dawn D. Matthews. 600 pages. 1999. 0-7808-0389-2. $78.

Domestic Violence & Child Abuse Sourcebook

Basic Information about Spousal/Partner, Child, and Elder Physical, Emotional, and Sexual Abuse, Teen Dating Violence, and Stalking, Including Information about Hotlines, Safe Houses, Safety Plans, and Other Resources for Support and Assistance, Community Initiatives, and Reports on Current Directions in Research and Treatment; Along with a Glossary, Sources for Further Reading, and Governmental and Non-Governmental Organizations Contact Information

Edited by Helene Henderson. 600 pages. 1999. 0-7808-0235-7. $78.

Ear, Nose & Throat Disorders Sourcebook

Basic Information about Disorders of the Ears, Nose, Sinus Cavities, Pharynx, and Larynx, Including Ear Infections, Tinnitus, Vestibular Disorders, Allergic and Non-Allergic Rhinitis, Sore Throats, Tonsillitis, and Cancers That Affect the Ears, Nose, Sinuses, and Throat, Along with Reports on Current Research Initiatives, a Glossary of Related Medical Terms, and a Directory of Sources for Further Help and Information

Edited by Karen Bellenir and Linda M. Shin. 576 pages. 1998. 0-7808-0206-3. $78.

"Overall, this sourcebook is helpful for the consumer seeking information on ENT issues. It is recommended for public libraries."
— *American Reference Books Annual, '99*

"Recent and recommended reference source."
— *Booklist, Dec '98*

Endocrine & Metabolic Disorders Sourcebook

Basic Information for the Layperson about Pancreatic and Insulin-Related Disorders Such as Pancreatitis, Diabetes, and Hypoglycemia; Adrenal Gland Disorders Such as Cushing's Syndrome, Addison's Disease, and Congenital Adrenal Hyperplasia; Pituitary Gland Disorders Such as Growth Hormone Deficiency, Acromegaly, and Pituitary Tumors; Thyroid Disorders Such as Hypothyroidism, Graves' Disease, Hashimoto's Disease, and Goiter; Hyperparathyroidism; and Other Diseases and Syndromes of Hormone Imbalance or Metabolic Dysfunction, Along with Reports on Current Research Initiatives

Edited by Linda M. Shin. 574 pages. 1998. 0-7808-0207-1. $78.

"Recent and recommended reference source."
— *Booklist, Dec '98*

Environmentally Induced Disorders Sourcebook

Basic Information about Diseases and Syndromes Linked to Exposure to Pollutants and Other Substances in Outdoor and Indoor Environments Such as Lead, Asbestos, Formaldehyde, Mercury, Emissions, Noise, and More

Edited by Allan R. Cook. 620 pages. 1997. 0-7808-0083-4. $78.

"Recent and recommended reference source."
— *Booklist, Sept '98*

"This book will be a useful addition to anyone's library."
— *Choice Health Sciences Supplement, May '98*

". . . a good survey of numerous environmentally induced physical disorders . . . a useful addition to anyone's library."
— *Doody's Health Science Book Reviews, Jan '98*

". . . provide[s] introductory information from the best authorities around. Since this volume covers topics that potentially affect everyone, it will surely be one of the most frequently consulted volumes in the *Health Reference Series*." — *Rettig on Reference, Nov '97*

Ethical Issues in Medicine Sourcebook

Basic Information about Controversial Treatment Issues, Genetic Research, Reproductive Technologies, and End-of-Life Decisions, Including Topics Such as Cloning, Abortion, Fertility Management, Organ Transplantation, Health Care Rationing, Advance Directives, Living Wills, Physician-Assisted Suicide, Euthanasia, and More; Along with a Glossary and Resources for Additional Information

Edited by Helene Henderson. 600 pages. 1999. 0-7808-0237-3. $78.

Fitness & Exercise Sourcebook

Basic Information on Fitness and Exercise, Including Fitness Activities for Specific Age Groups, Exercise for People with Specific Medical Conditions, How to Begin a Fitness Program in Running, Walking, Swimming, Cycling, and Other Athletic Activities, and Recent Research in Fitness and Exercise

Edited by Dan R. Harris. 663 pages. 1996. 0-7808-0186-5. $78.

"A good resource for general readers."
— *Choice, Nov '97*

"The perennial popularity of the topic . . . make this an appealing selection for public libraries."
— *Rettig on Reference, Jun/Jul '97*

Food & Animal Borne Diseases Sourcebook

Basic Information about Diseases That Can Be Spread to Humans through the Ingestion of Contaminated Food or Water or by Contact with Infected Animals and Insects, Such as Botulism, E. Coli, Hepatitis A, Trichinosis, Lyme Disease, and Rabies, Along with Information Regarding Prevention and Treatment Methods, and a Special Section for International Travelers Describing Diseases Such as Cholera, Malaria, Travelers' Diarrhea, and Yellow Fever, and Offering Recommendations for Avoiding Illness

Edited by Karen Bellenir and Peter D. Dresser. 535 pages. 1995. 0-7808-0033-8. $78.

"Targeting general readers and providing them with a single, comprehensive source of information on selected topics, this book continues, with the excellent caliber of its predecessors, to catalog topical information on health matters of general interest. Readable and thorough, this valuable resource is highly recommended for all libraries."
— *Academic Library Book Review, Summer '96*

"A comprehensive collection of authoritative information." — *Emergency Medical Services, Oct '95*

Food Safety Sourcebook

Basic Consumer Health Information about the Safe Handling of Meat, Poultry, Seafood, Eggs, Fruit Juices, and Other Food Items, and Facts about Pesticides, Drinking Water, Food Safety Overseas, and the Onset, Duration, and Symptoms of Foodborne Illnesses, Including Types of Pathogenic Bacteria, Parasitic Protozoa, Worms, Viruses, and Natural Toxins; Along with the Role of the Consumer, the Food Handler, and the Government in Food Safety; a Glossary, and Resources for Additional Help and Information

Edited by Dawn D. Matthews. 339 pages. 1999. 0-7808-0326-4. $48.

Forensic Medicine Sourcebook

Basic Consumer Information for the Layperson about Forensic Medicine, Including Crime Scene Investigation, Evidence Collection and Analysis, Expert Testimony, Computer-Aided Criminal Identification, Digital Imaging in the Courtroom, DNA Profiling, Accident Reconstruction, Autopsies, Ballistics, Drugs and Explosives Detection, Latent Fingerprints, Product Tampering, and Questioned Document Examination; Along with Statistical Data, a Glossary of Forensics Terminology, and Listings of Sources for Further Help and Information

Edited by Annemarie S. Muth. 574 pages. 1999. 0-7808-0232-2. $78.

Gastrointestinal Diseases & Disorders Sourcebook

Basic Information about Gastroesophageal Reflux Disease (Heartburn), Ulcers, Diverticulosis, Irritable Bowel Syndrome, Crohn's Disease, Ulcerative Colitis, Diarrhea, Constipation, Lactose Intolerance, Hemorrhoids, Hepatitis, Cirrhosis, and Other Digestive Problems, Featuring Statistics, Descriptions of Symptoms, and Current Treatment Methods of Interest for Persons Living with Upper and Lower Gastrointestinal Maladies

Edited by Linda M. Ross. 413 pages. 1996. 0 7808-0078-8. $78.

"... very readable form. The successful editorial work that brought this material together into a useful and understandable reference makes accessible to all readers information that can help them more effectively understand and obtain help for digestive tract problems." — *Choice, Feb '97*

Genetic Disorders Sourcebook

Basic Information about Heritable Diseases and Disorders Such as Down Syndrome, PKU, Hemophilia, Von Willebrand Disease, Gaucher Disease, Tay-Sachs Disease, and Sickle-Cell Disease, Along with Information about Genetic Screening, Gene Therapy, Home Care, and Including Source Listings for Further Help and Information on More Than 300 Disorders

Edited by Karen Bellenir. 642 pages. 1996. 0-7808-0034-6. $78.

"Provides essential medical information to both the general public and those diagnosed with a serious or fatal genetic disease or disorder." — *Choice, Jan '97*

"Geared toward the lay public. It would be well placed in all public libraries and in those hospital and medical libraries in which access to genetic references is limited." — *Doody's Health Sciences Book Review, Oct '96*

Head Trauma Sourcebook

Basic Information for the Layperson about Open-Head and Closed-Head Injuries, Treatment Advances, Recovery, and Rehabilitation, Along with Reports on Current Research Initiatives

Edited by Karen Bellenir. 414 pages. 1997. 0-7808-0208-X. $78.

Health Insurance Sourcebook

Basic Information about Managed Care Organizations, Traditional Fee-for-Service Insurance, Insurance Portability and Pre-Existing Conditions Clauses, Medicare, Medicaid, Social Security, and Military Health Care, Along with Information about Insurance Fraud

Edited by Wendy Wilcox. 530 pages. 1997. 0-7808-0222-5. $78.

"Particularly useful because it brings much of this information together in one volume." — *Medical Reference Services Quarterly, Fall '98*

"The layout of the book is particularly helpful as it provides easy access to reference material. A most useful addition to the vast amount of information about health insurance. The use of data from U.S. government agencies is most commendable. Useful in a library or learning center for healthcare professional students." — *Doody's Health Sciences Book Reviews, Nov '97*

Healthy Aging Sourcebook

Basic Consumer Health Information about Maintaining Health through the Aging Process, Including Advice on Nutrition, Exercise, and Sleep, Help in Making Decisions about Midlife Issues and Retirement, and Guidance Concerning Practical and Informed Choices in Health Consumerism; Along with Data Concerning the Theories of Aging, Different Experiences in Aging by Minority Groups, and Facts about Aging Now and Aging in the Future; and Featuring a Glossary, a Guide to Consumer Help, Additional Suggested Reading, and Practical Resource Directory

Edited by Jenifer Swanson. 536 pages. 1999. 0-7808-0390-6. $78.

Heart Diseases & Disorders Sourcebook, 2nd edition

Basic Consumer Health Information about Heart Attacks, Angina, Rhythm Disorders, Heart Failure, Valve Disease, Congenital Heart Disorders, and More, Including Descriptions of Surgical Procedures and Other Interventions, Medications, Cardiac Rehabilitation, Risk Identification, and Prevention Tips; Along with Statistical Data, Reports on Current Research Initiatives, a Glossary of Cardiovascular Terms, and Resource Directory

Edited by Karen Bellenir. 600 pages. 1999. 0-7808-0238-1. $78.

Immune System Disorders Sourcebook

Basic Information about Lupus, Multiple Sclerosis, Guillain-Barré Syndrome, Chronic Granulomatous Disease, and More, Along with Statistical and Demographic Data and Reports on Current Research Initiatives

Edited by Allan R. Cook. 608 pages. 1997. 0-7808-0209-8. $78.

Infant & Toddler Health Sourcebook

Basic Consumer Health Information about the Physical and Mental Development of Newborns, Infants, and Toddlers, Including Neonatal Concerns, Nutritional Recommendations, Immunization Schedules, Common Pediatric Disorders, Assessments and Milestones, Safety Tips, and Advice for Parents and Other Caregivers; Along with a Glossary of Terms and Resource Listings for Additional Help

Edited by Jenifer Swanson. 600 pages. 1999. 0-7808-0246-2. $78.

Kidney & Urinary Tract Diseases & Disorders Sourcebook

Basic Information about Kidney Stones, Urinary Incontinence, Bladder Disease, End Stage Renal Disease, Dialysis, and More, Along with Statistical and Demographic Data and Reports on Current Research Initiatives

Edited by Linda M. Ross. 602 pages. 1997. 0-7808-0079-6. $78.

Learning Disabilities Sourcebook

Basic Information about Disorders Such as Dyslexia, Visual and Auditory Processing Deficits, Attention Deficit/Hyperactivity Disorder, and Autism, Along with Statistical and Demographic Data, Reports on Current Research Initiatives, an Explanation of the Assessment Process, and a Special Section for Adults with Learning Disabilities

Edited by Linda M. Shin. 579 pages. 1998. 0-7808-0210-1. $78.

"Readable . . . provides a solid base of information regarding successful techniques used with individuals who have learning disabilities, as well as practical suggestions for educators and family members. Clear language, concise descriptions, and pertinent information for contacting multiple resources add to the strength of this book as a useful tool." — *Choice, Feb '99*

"Recent and recommended reference source."
— *Booklist, Sept '98*

Liver Disorders Sourcebook

Basic Consumer Health Information about the Liver and How It Works; Liver Diseases, Including Cancer, Cirrhosis, Hepatitis, and Toxic and Drug Related Diseases; Tips for Maintaining a Healthy Liver; Laboratory Tests, Radiology Tests, and Facts about Liver Transplantation; Along with a Section on Support Groups, a Glossary, and Resource Listings

Edited by Joyce Brennfleck Shannon. 600 pages. 1999. 0-7808-0383-3. $78.

Medical Tests Sourcebook

Basic Consumer Health Information about Medical Tests, Including Periodic Health Exams, General Screening Tests, Tests You Can Do at Home, Findings of the U.S. Preventive Services Task Force, X-ray and Radiology Tests, Electrical Tests, Tests of Blood and Other Body Fluids and Tissues, Scope Tests, Lung Tests, Genetic Tests, Pregnancy Tests, Newborn Screening Tests, Sexually Transmitted Disease Tests, and Computer Aided Diagnoses; Along with a Section on Paying for Medical Tests, a Glossary, and Resource Listings

Edited by Joyce Brennfleck Shannon. 691 pages. 1999. 0-7808-0243-8. $78.

Men's Health Concerns Sourcebook

Basic Information about Health Issues That Affect Men, Featuring Facts about the Top Causes of Death in Men, Including Heart Disease, Stroke, Cancers, Prostate Disorders, Chronic Obstructive Pulmonary Disease, Pneumonia and Influenza, Human Immunodeficiency Virus and Acquired Immune Deficiency Syndrome, Diabetes Mellitus, Stress, Suicide, Accidents and Homicides; and Facts about Common Concerns for Men, Including Impotence, Contraception, Circumcision, Sleep Disorders, Snoring, Hair Loss, Diet, Nutrition, Exercise, Kidney and Urological Disorders, and Backaches

Edited by Allan R. Cook. 738 pages. 1998. 0-7808-0212-8. $78.

"Recent and recommended reference source."
— *Booklist, Dec '98*

Mental Health Disorders Sourcebook, 1st Edition

Basic Information about Schizophrenia, Depression, Bipolar Disorder, Panic Disorder, Obsessive-Compulsive Disorder, Phobias and Other Anxiety Disorders, Paranoia and Other Personality Disorders, Eating Disorders, and Sleep Disorders, Along with Information about Treatment and Therapies

Edited by Karen Bellenir. 548 pages. 1995. 0-7808-0040-0. $78.

"This is an excellent new book . . . written in easy-to-understand language."
— *Booklist Health Science Supplement, Oct '97*

". . . useful for public and academic libraries and consumer health collections."
— *Medical Reference Services Quarterly, Spring '97*

"The great strengths of the book are its readability and its inclusion of places to find more information. Especially recommended." — *RQ, Winter '96*

". . . a good resource for a consumer health library."
— *Bulletin of the MLA, Oct '96*

Mental Health Disorders Sourcebook, 2nd Edition

Basic Consumer Health Information about Anxiety Disorders, Depression and Other Mood Disorders, Eating Disorders, Personality Disorders, Schizophrenia, and More, Including Disease Descriptions, Treatment Options, and Reports on Current Research Initiatives; Along with Statistical Data, Tips for Maintaining Mental Health, a Glossary, and Directory of Sources for Additional Help and Information

Edited by Karen Bellenir. 600 pages. 1999. 0-7808-0240-3. $78.

Ophthalmic Disorders Sourcebook

Basic Information about Glaucoma, Cataracts, Macular Degeneration, Strabismus, Refractive Disorders, and More, Along with Statistical and Demographic Data and Reports on Current Research Initiatives

Edited by Linda M. Ross. 631 pages. 1996. 0-7808-0081-8. $78.

Oral Health Sourcebook

Basic Information about Diseases and Conditions Affecting Oral Health, Including Cavities, Gum Disease, Dry Mouth, Oral Cancers, Fever Blisters, Canker Sores, Oral Thrush, Bad Breath, Temporomandibular Disorders, and other Craniofacial Syndromes, Along with Statistical Data on the Oral Health of Americans, Oral Hygiene, Emergency First Aid, Information on Treatment Procedures and Methods of Replacing Lost Teeth

Edited by Allan R. Cook. 558 pages. 1997. 0-7808-0082-6. $78.

Osteoporosis Sourcebook

Basic Consumer Health Information about Primary and Secondary Osteoporosis, Juvenile Osteoporosis, Related Conditions, and Other Such Bone Disorders as Fibrous Dysplasia, Myeloma, Osteogenesis Imperfecta, Osteopetrosis, and Paget's Disease; Along with Information about Risk Factors, Treatments, Traditional and Non-Traditional Pain Management, and Including a Glossary and Resource Directory

Edited by Allan R. Cook. 600 pages. 1999. 0-7808-0239-X. $78.

Pain Sourcebook

Basic Information about Specific Forms of Acute and Chronic Pain, Including Headaches, Back Pain, Muscular Pain, Neuralgia, Surgical Pain, and Cancer Pain, Along with Pain Relief Options Such as Analgesics, Narcotics, Nerve Blocks, Transcutaneous Nerve Stimulation, and Alternative Forms of Pain Control, Including Biofeedback, Imaging, Behavior Modification, and Relaxation Techniques

Edited by Allan R. Cook. 667 pages. 1997. 0-7808-0213-6. $78.

Pediatric Cancer Sourcebook

Basic Consumer Health Information about Leukemias, Brain Tumors, Sarcomas, Lymphomas, and Other Cancers in Infants, Children, and Adolescents, Including Descriptions of Cancers, Treatments, and Coping Strategies; Along with Suggestions for Parents, Caregivers, and Concerned Relatives, a Glossary of Cancer Terms, and Resource Listings

Edited by Edward J. Prucha. 587 pages. 1999. 0-7808-0245-4. $78.

Physical & Mental Issues in Aging Sourcebook

Basic Consumer Health Information on Physical and Mental Disorders Associated with the Aging Process, Including Concerns about Cardiovascular Disease, Pulmonary Disease, Oral Health, Digestive Disorders, Musculoskeletal and Skin Disorders, Metabolic Changes, Sexual and Reproductive Issues, and Changes in Vision, Hearing, and Other Senses; Along with Data about Longevity and Causes of Death, Information on Acute and Chronic Pain, Descriptions of Mental Concerns, a Glossary of Terms, and Resource Listings for Additional Help

Edited by Jenifer Swanson. 660 pages. 1999. 0-7808-0233-0. $78.

Pregnancy & Birth Sourcebook

Basic Information about Planning for Pregnancy, Maternal Health, Fetal Growth and Development, Labor and Delivery, Postpartum and Perinatal Care, Pregnancy in Mothers with Special Concerns, and Disorders of Pregnancy, Including Genetic Counseling, Nutrition and Exercise, Obstetrical Tests, Pregnancy Discomfort, Multiple Births, Cesarean Sections, Medical Testing of Newborns, Breastfeeding, Gestational Diabetes, and Ectopic Pregnancy

Edited by Heather E. Aldred. 737 pages. 1997. 0-7808-0216-0. $78.

"A well-organized handbook. Recommended."
— Choice, Apr '98

"Recent and recommended reference source."
— Booklist, Mar '98

"Recommended for public libraries."
— American Reference Books Annual, '98

Public Health Sourcebook

Basic Information about Government Health Agencies, Including National Health Statistics and Trends, Healthy People 2000 Program Goals and Objectives, the Centers for Disease Control and Prevention, the Food and Drug Administration, and the National Institutes of Health, Along with Full Contact Information for Each Agency

Edited by Wendy Wilcox. 698 pages. 1998. 0-7808-0220-9. $78.

"Recent and recommended reference source."
— Booklist, Sept '98

"This consumer guide provides welcome assistance in navigating the maze of federal health agencies and their data on public health concerns."
— SciTech Book News, Sept '98

Rehabilitation Sourcebook

Basic Consumer Health Information about Rehabilitation for People Recovering from Heart Surgery, Spinal Cord Injury, Stroke, Orthopedic Impairments, Amputation, Pulmonary Impairments, Traumatic Injury, and More, Including Physical Therapy, Occupational Therapy, Speech/Language Therapy, Massage Therapy, Dance Therapy, Art Therapy, and Recreational Therapy; Along with Information on Assistive and Adaptive Devices, a Glossary, and Resources for Additional Help and Information

Edited by Dawn D. Matthews. 531 pages. 1999. 0-7808-0236-5. $78.

Respiratory Diseases & Disorders Sourcebook

Basic Information about Respiratory Diseases and Disorders, Including Asthma, Cystic Fibrosis, Pneumonia, the Common Cold, Influenza, and Others, Featuring Facts about the Respiratory System, Statistical and Demographic Data, Treatments, Self-Help Management Suggestions, and Current Research Initiatives

Edited by Allan R. Cook and Peter D. Dresser. 771 pages. 1995. 0-7808-0037-0. $78.

"Designed for the layperson and for patients and their families coping with respiratory illness. . . . an extensive array of information on diagnosis, treatment, management, and prevention of respiratory illnesses for the general reader."
— Choice, Jun '96

"A highly recommended text for all collections. It is a comforting reminder of the power of knowledge that good books carry between their covers."
— Academic Library Book Review, Spring '96

"This sourcebook offers a comprehensive collection of authoritative information presented in a nontechnical, humanitarian style for patients, families, and caregivers."
— Association of Operating Room Nurses, Sept/Oct '95

Sexually Transmitted Diseases Sourcebook

Basic Information about Herpes, Chlamydia, Gonorrhea, Hepatitis, Nongonoccocal Urethritis, Pelvic Inflammatory Disease, Syphilis, AIDS, and More, Along with Current Data on Treatments and Preventions

Edited by Linda M. Ross. 550 pages. 1997. 0-7808-0217-9. $78.

Skin Disorders Sourcebook

Basic Information about Common Skin and Scalp Conditions Caused by Aging, Allergies, Immune Reactions, Sun Exposure, Infectious Organisms, Parasites, Cosmetics, and Skin Traumas, Including Abrasions, Cuts, and Pressure Sores, Along with Information on Prevention and Treatment

Edited by Allan R. Cook. 647 pages. 1997. 0-7808-0080-X. $78.

". . . comprehensive easily read reference book."
— *Doody's Health Sciences Book Reviews, Oct '97*

Sleep Disorders Sourcebook

Basic Consumer Health Information about Sleep and Its Disorders, Including Insomnia, Sleepwalking, Sleep Apnea, Restless Leg Syndrome, and Narcolepsy; Along with Data about Shiftwork and Its Effects, Information on the Societal Costs of Sleep Deprivation, Descriptions of Treatment Options, a Glossary of Terms, and Resource Listings for Additional Help

Edited by Jenifer Swanson. 439 pages. 1998. 0-7808-0234-9. $78.

"Recent and recommended reference source."
— *Booklist, Feb '99*

Sports Injuries Sourcebook

Basic Consumer Health Information about Common Sports Injuries, Prevention of Injury in Specific Sports, Tips for Training, and Rehabilitation from Injury; Along with Information about Special Concerns for Children, Young Girls in Athletic Training Programs, Senior Athletes, and Women Athletes, and a Directory of Resources for Further Help and Information

Edited by Heather E. Aldred. 624 pages. 1999. 0-7808-0218-7. $78.

Substance Abuse Sourcebook

Basic Health-Related Information about the Abuse of Legal and Illegal Substances Such as Alcohol, Tobacco, Prescription Drugs, Marijuana, Cocaine, and Heroin; and Including Facts about Substance Abuse Prevention Strategies, Intervention Methods, Treatment and Recovery Programs, and a Section Addressing the Special Problems Related to Substance Abuse during Pregnancy

Edited by Karen Bellenir. 573 pages. 1996. 0-7808-0038-9. $78.

"A valuable addition to any health reference section. Highly recommended."
— *The Book Report, Mar/Apr '97*

". . . a comprehensive collection of substance abuse information that's both highly readable and compact. Families and caregivers of substance abusers will find the information enlightening and helpful, while teachers, social workers and journalists should benefit from the concise format. Recommended."
— *Drug Abuse Update, Winter '96-'97*

Women's Health Concerns Sourcebook

Basic Information about Health Issues That Affect Women, Featuring Facts about Menstruation and Other Gynecological Concerns, Including Endometriosis, Fibroids, Menopause, and Vaginitis; Reproductive Concerns, Including Birth Control, Infertility, and Abortion; and Facts about Additional Physical, Emotional, and Mental Health Concerns Prevalent among Women Such as Osteoporosis, Urinary Tract Disorders, Eating Disorders, and Depression, Along with Tips for Maintaining a Healthy Lifestyle

Edited by Heather Aldred. 567 pages. 1997. 0-7808-0219-5. $78.

"Handy compilation. There is an impressive range of diseases, devices, disorders, procedures, and other physical and emotional issues covered . . . well organized, illustrated, and indexed."
— *Choice, Jan '98*

Workplace Health & Safety Sourcebook

Basic Information about Musculoskeletal Injuries, Cumulative Trauma Disorders, Occupational Carcinogens and Other Toxic Materials, Child Labor, Workplace Violence, Histoplasmosis, Transmission of HIV and Hepatitis-B Viruses, and Occupational Hazards Associated with Various Industries, Including Mining, Confined Spaces, Agriculture, Construction, Electrical Work, and the Medical Professions, with Information on Mortality and Other Statistical Data, Preventative Measures, Reproductive Risks, Reducing Stress for Shiftworkers, Noise Hazards, Industrial Back Belts, Reducing Contamination at Home, Preventing Allergic Reactions to Rubber Latex, and More; Along with Public and Private Programs and Initiatives, a Glossary, and Sources for Additional Help and Information

Edited by Helene Henderson. 600 pages. 1999. 0-7808-0231-4. $78.

Health Reference Series Cumulative Index

A Comprehensive Index to 42 Volumes of the Health Reference Series, 1990-1998

1,500 pages. 1999. 0-7808-0382-5. $78.